TRANSMISSIBLE DISEASES AND BLOOD TRANSFUSION

DEVELOPMENTS IN HEMATOLOGY AND IMMUNOLOGY

Volume 37

The titles published in this series are listed at the end of this volume.

Transmissible Diseases and Blood Transfusion

Proceedings of the Twenty-Sixth International Symposium on Blood Transfusion, Groningen, NL,
Organized by the Sanquin Division Blood Bank Noord Nederland

edited by

C. TH. SMIT SIBINGA
Blood Bank Noord Nederland,
Groningen, The Netherlands

and

R. Y. DODD
ARC Jerome Holland Laboratory,
Rockville, MD, U.S.A.

KLUWER ACADEMIC PUBLISHERS
DORDRECHT / BOSTON / LONDON

A C.I.P. Catalogue record for this book is available from the Library of Congress

ISBN 978-1-4419-5233-2

Published by Kluwer Academic Publishers,
P.O. Box 17, 3300 AA Dordrecht, The Netherlands.

Sold and distributed in North, Central and South America
by Kluwer Academic Publishers,
101 Philip Drive, Norwell, MA 02061, U.S.A.

In all other countries, sold and distributed
by Kluwer Academic Publishers,
P.O. Box 322, 3300 AH Dordrecht, The Netherlands.

Printed on acid-free paper

This 26th Sanquin International Symposium on Blood Transfusion was supported by WHO and conducted under the auspices of the Sanquin Blood Supply Foundation.

Baxter

Acknowledgement

This publication has been made possible through the support of Baxter, which is gratefully acknowledged.

CONTENTS

III. TRANSMISSIBLE DISEASES

IV. PREVENTATIVE ASPECTS

MODERATORS AND SPEAKERS

Moderators

R.Y. Dodd (chairman)	–	American Red Cross Jerome Holland Laboratory, Rockville, MD, USA
J.H. Marcelis	–	Sanquin Division Blood Bank de Meijerij, Eindhoven, NL
C.L. van der Poel	–	Sanquin Blood Supply Foundation, Amsterdam, NL
C.Th. Smit Sibinga	–	Sanquin Consulting Service, Groningen, NL
S.L. Stramer	–	National Testing and Reference Laboratory and Blood Services American Red Cross, Gaithersburg, MD, USA
D.S. Wages	-	Cerus Corporation, Concord, CA, USA
H.J.C. de Wit	-	Sanquin Blood Supply Foundation, Amsterdam, NL

Speakers

H.T.M. Cuypers	–	Sanquin Blood Supply Foundation, Division CLB Diagnositics, Amsterdam, NL
L.M. Kortbeek	–	RIVM, Bilthoven, NL
D. Leiby	–	American Red Cross Jerome Holland Institute, Rockville, MD, USA
P.W.J. Peters	–	Professor of Teratology, University Medical Centre Utrecht, Utrecht, NL Chief Inspector Food, Inspectorate for Health Protection and Veterinary Public Health, 's-Gravenhage, NL
E. Pinelli	–	RIVM, Bilthoven, NL
M.J. Postma	–	University of Groningen Institute for Drug Exploration (GUIDE), Groningen, NL

E.J. Ruitenberg	–	Sanquin Blood Supply Foundation, Divison CLB, Amsterdam, NL
G.P.A. Smit	–	Beatrix Children's Hospital, Groningen, NL
W.P.A. van der Tuuk Adriani	–	Sanquin Blood Supply Foundation, Division Blood Bank Noord Nederland, Groningen, NL
M.L. Turner	–	Edinburgh & S.E. Scotland BTS, Edinburgh, UK
G. Vercauteren	–	WHO BSCT, Geneva, CH
J.Th.M. de Wolf	–	Clinical Haematologist, University Hospital Groningen, Groningen, NL

OPENING ADDRESS

A very warm welcome to you all. Due to the 11 September event travelling might have been difficult and many people decided not to go to congresses these days. Many congresses have been cancelled. So, I am very happy to see you all here, because I think that the programme of this 26th SANQUIN International Symposium on Blood Transfusion presented is very promising. Blood transfusion and quality of blood transfusion supports many people in the world, also victims of violence as we have experienced these last weeks. It is therefore good to continue along the line and have this symposium. Although the programme was planned two years ago, it is very timely especially in relation to Europe and the European Directive that is now prepared in the European Parliament in Brussels. When I was informed that Prof. Douglas Starr could not be here, I decided to do two things. By fortune I got access to some beautiful material that illustrates some small but dominant and important events in history of blood transfusion as a whole, but perhaps more specifically in the Netherlands. These events have influenced the Western world and blood transfusion therefore as a whole. It is the pictorial history of 25 years pioneering in blood transfusion, the career of Dr. Cees Smit Sibinga, the organiser of these International Symposia on Blood Transfusion that have taken place uninterruptedly since 1976.

Many of the issues to be discussed during this symposium relate to safety of blood in that part of the blood transfusion chain that is the responsibility of blood supply organisations. One of the main issues now is paid versus non-paid, remunerated versus non-remunerated donation. which is not only an ethical issue but also a safety issue. What will be indicated in the Directive is that there is one major issue: Safety First. Common standards for safety throughout the European Union and 'safety' first bring me to the thought that where blood supply systems in Europe - in the Western world - have proven to be able to achieve adequate sufficiency with non-remunerated donations, it would be a threat when paid donation would be allowed. Those systems that rely on the non-remunerated donor might be disturbed by allowing organisations that use paid donors to penetrate into the country and into the donor population. That weighs heavier than the fear that with anchoring non-remunerated donation in the European Directive there might be the chance of not having adequate supply especially in plasma products. The problem of disturbing the non-remunerated donor system is more severe. So, if you think of safety first and look into donor populations, non-remunerated donations should be THE choice throughout

Europe. The same can be said about virus testing and virus inactivation. Of the amendments that have been accepted now by European Parliament, there is one that says that techniques for virus inactivation should be implemented as soon as they become available. This means that the discussion about optimal safety versus maximal safety - about cost per case prevented and quality adjusted life saved, can be concluded. The indication 'implement as soon as possible' is driven by the legislation in the European Union, especially product liability and the way to deal with products in terms of being producers of blood products. If you want to achieve a common level of safety, the way to handle these techniques and to introduce these techniques should be co-ordinated. That prevents us from going in different directions in countries that are so alike like countries within the European Union. Although we are aware of the fact that common standards tend to be absolute standards and although the influence of product liability is high, we realise that the difference between Western industrialised countries and Eastern developing countries might grow bigger. That is why it is good that this symposium also includes a presentation about how to implement quality management throughout the world. With introducing quality management and blood supply systems on a national level we can come to comparable safety for patients needing blood and blood transfusion.

This is in more than one aspect a special symposium.

First, Dr. Cees Smit Sibinga is no more the director of the Blood Bank Noord Nederland. Mid September we had a farewell symposium thanking him for all he had done. At that symposium we announced that there would be a comeback and we have seen the first comeback of Cees Smit Sibinga being the head of the SANQUIN Consulting Service. In this role he will advice – sometimes with a WHO hat on – different countries in structuring blood supply systems and implementing quality systems and management.

Second, Dr. Cees Smit Sibinga will remain the organiser of these symposia. I would like to thank him and all the people behind the organisation for doing so. Again this programme is very promising and I hope that the discussions that we will have will be the basis for scientific evidence fundamental to common safety standards that should be implemented in EU Directive and other international standards for blood and blood transfusion. Thank you, I hope that this will be a good congress to you all.

H.J.C. de Wit,
Board of Directors, SANQUIN Blood Supply Foundation
Amsterdam, NL

I. BLOOD SAFETY ASPECTS

GERMS, GELS AND GENOMES. A PERSONAL RECOLLECTION OF 30 YEARS IN BLOOD SAFETY TESTING

Roger Y. Dodd[1]

Introduction

Thirty years ago, there was but one test to assure the microbiological safety of the blood supply. This was accompanied by a donor questionnaire that focussed on a history of hepatitis, intravenous drug use and international travel. Today, we use 8 to 10 separate tests, designed to detect 12 different infection markers, and the latest version of the uniform donor questionnaire has no less that 32 separate questions (some of which are themselves multi-part), with more waiting in the wings. Over this period, philosophies have changed and cries for increased blood safety have now been replaced by petitions for financial relief to pay for increased blood safety measures. In this chapter, I will retrace some of this history of blood safety, with special reference to test methods. In parallel, I will consider the evolution of decision-making in this area, and will end by questioning the extent to which we, as blood bankers, may have become trapped in our own history.

Table 1 indicates the timeline of introduction of blood donor screening tests and their principal modifications in the USA. It is key to note that, once a test for a marker has been introduced, it has only been withdrawn as a result of the introduction of an improved version of the test for that marker. There is no question that the use of these tests, along with careful measures to select donor populations, had a profound impact on blood safety. Table 2 defines current incidence and prevalence rates for key markers in the Red Cross voluntary donor population, and compares these rates with those for the US population overall.

Syphilis and hepatitis: the early days

Testing for syphilis was the first laboratory measure to be applied to the microbiological safety of blood for transfusion. This was presumably prompted by recognized instances of transfusion syphilis, and remains with us after more than half a century, even though the efficacy of this measure (if any) is unknown. Lew Barker, writing in 1984, reviewed the social history of the introduction of donor syphilis testing, finding it to be quite unremarkable and completely de

1. Head, Transmissible Diseases Department, American Red Cross Holland Laboratory 15601 Crabbs Branch Way, Rockville MD 20855, USA. dodd@usa.redcross.org.

Table 1. Timeline for introduction of blood donor screening tests, USA

Year	Marker	Technology
1940s	Syphilis	Reagin-based tests
1970-72	HBsAG	Gel precipitation
1972-4	HBsAG	Second generation (CEP, Rheophoresis, RPHA)
1974	HBsAG	RIA
1979-80	HBsAG	EIA*
1985	anti-HIV	EIA
1986-87	ALT	Enzymatic
1986-87	anti-HBc	EIA*
1988	anti-HTLV-I	EIA
1990	anti HCV 1.0	EIA
1992	anti HCV 2.0	EIA
1992	anti HIV-1/HIV-2	EIA*
1995	Syphilis	TPHA*
1996	HIV-1 p24	EIA*
1996	anti HCV 3.0	EIA*
1998	anti HTLV I/II	EIA*
1999	HCV RNA	PCR/TMA*
2000	HIV RNA	PCR/TMA*

* Tests in current use (June, 2000).

Table 2: Incidence and prevalence of key infection markers among American Red Cross blood donors, 1999, compared to rates for the US population [37]

Agent	Prevalence* (donors)	Prevalence (US, overall)	Incidence† (Donors)	Incidence (US, overall)
HBV (HBsAg)	84.4	NA	4.5‡	114.4
HCV	386.3	1800	2.8	13.4
HIV	11.8	136	1.7	15

* Prevalence per hundred thousand first-time blood donors.
† Incidence per hundred thousand person-years among repeat donors.
‡ Corrected for transient nature of HBsAg [28].

void of the turmoil associated with the introduction of testing for antibodies to HIV [1]. The original reagin-base serologic tests for syphilis, despite their obvious failings in terms of sensitivity and specificity, continued in wide use until the mid 1990s, until replaced by treponemal tests. I will return to this topic later.

Almost from the outset, viral hepatitis was recognized as the most frequent, and serious infectious outcome of blood transfusion. Figures vary, but the remarkable studies of J. Garrot Allen in the 1960s, revealed that at least 1.5% of transfused patients developed overt, acute, symptomatic hepatitis [2]. Studies that relied upon sensitive measures of liver damage were even more ominous, with frequencies of posttransfusion liver dysfunction as high as 30%. These findings were clearly linked to the epidemiological background of the implicated donors, with paid and imprisoned donors providing the greatest risk. In the early 1960s, the virology of hepatitis proved intractable. Two types of hepatitis were recognized on epidemiologic grounds and controversial, but groundbreaking studies by Krugman did show that the so called "serum" and "infectious" hepatitides were caused by clearly separable infectious agents [3]. In the absence of any definitive serology, however, there was no direct means to assure that blood donors did not carry the infectious agent(s) of hepatitis. Two measures were, however, implemented: exclusion of donors with a history of viral hepatitis, on the assumption that such individuals could still be infected and infectious, and a move to eliminate paid and prison donations. There is little doubt that the second of these had a tremendous impact upon the incidence of post-transfusion infection and studies suggest that a significant proportion of donors with a history of hepatitis showed evidence of past (and potentially continuing) infection with hepatitis B virus (HBV) and/or hepatitis C virus (HCV) [4].

During the early 1960s, there were also a number of proposals to test blood donors for markers of liver dysfunction. At that time, tests were poorly characterized and, although strangely prescient, these proposals were not widely adopted. In terms of the broader decision process, it is probably fair to say that physicians, researchers, policymakers and the public were all strongly committed to an outcome that would reduce, or eliminate the risk of transfusion hepatitis. Nevertheless, the concept of hepatitis risk was so ingrained that this disease was considered to be an inevitable consequence of transfusion medicine and almost all States enacted blood shield laws to protect transfusionists from medico-legal liability. It is hard to conceive that any such approach would be contemplated today!

Barry Blumberg's essentially serendipitous discovery of "Australia Antigen" (HBsAg) and its subsequent linkage to one form of viral hepatitis can be considered the first seminal event in the development of modern blood donor screening procedures and policies [5,6]. Not only was HBsAg clearly associated with what was then known as hepatitis B, but some studies had established that blood that was positive for the antigen clearly transmitted hepatitis B to recipients [7]. Test methods became available around 1969, but were not uniformly adopted until about 1970 or 1971. The very first test to be implemented was, almost unbelievably, Ouchterlony agar gel diffusion (AGD), using human or animal antibodies to detect the antigen in donor serum. It is important to recognize, however, that the actual level of HBsAg in a highly infectious sample was extraordinarily high – perhaps tens to hundreds of micrograms/mL. The AGD test was soon replaced by directed immunoprecipitation systems, such as counterimmunoelectrophoresis or rheophoresis in which an electrical potential or evaporative buffer flow forced the antibodies and antigen together, thus increasing speed and sensitivity. The tests were, however, highly subjective. Some alternative methods, such as reversed passive hemagglutination, were also developed and achieved a limited degree of implementation. Another historical footnote is that AGD was (retrospectively) defined as a "first generation" test and the agglutination and directed immunoprecipitation tests were defined as "second generation".

C.M. Ling and Lacey Overby, working at Abbott Laboratories, soon developed a tube-based, solid phase radioimmunoassay (RIA) for the detection of HBsAg [8]. This method clearly had greatly increased analytical sensitivity (e.g. around 1 ng/mL) relative to second generation tests and was formally defined as a "third generation" test. It was not long before the Bureau of Biologics (the then equivalent of the FDA) published a notice in the Federal Register, indicating that licensure of this third generation test was imminent and "advising" blood establishments to "become familiar" with it. Again foreshadowing the future, many blood bankers were heard to mutter comments like "we'll never be able to implement that technology in the blood bank environment". It was certainly a major challenge, but it was successfully accomplished.

At the time of implementation of RIA, it was widely anticipated that the problem of post-transfusion hepatitis would be solved. It had already been recognized that second generation tests did not eliminate all post-transfusion hepatitis – indeed, there was only about a 20% decline in reporting rates. However, by what turned out to be a bizarre coincidence, RIA generated about fivefold more reactive results that did the second-generation tests. It soon became apparent that most of the additional "detections" represented false-positives. This finding was a disappointment, but led directly to the introduction of additional confirmatory tests, and an enhanced perception of the rights of the donor to be properly informed about the significance of screening test results. After a relatively short time, RIA was replaced by enzyme immunoassay.

The problem of non-A, non-B hepatitis: days of confusion

The continuation of post-transfusion hepatitis remained a concern, but became an enigma when Robert Purcell and his colleagues at the NIH identified the hepatitis A virus (HAV) and developed serologic tests for it. Application of these tests to samples from the residual post-transfusion hepatitis cases showed that they were not due to infection with either HBV or HAV [9], leading to an almost 15-year search for the causative agent. The residual disease was termed non-A, non-B hepatitis (NANBH) and a number of important, large scale studies were initiated to characterize the disease and its transmission, and perhaps to develop an immunologic test. The latter effort was unsuccessful for many years, as witnessed by Harvey Alter's final score on attempts to apply candidate tests to his invaluable collection of samples: "viruses 11, investigators 0". What did emerge was a clear perspective on the incidence of the disease, and the identification of two donor markers that were able to predict increased risk for transmission of NANBH. One was an elevated level of alanine aminotransferase (ALT), the other was the presence of antibodies to the hepatitis B core antigen (anti-HBc) [10-13]. Neither was sensitive or specific, but it was anticipated that, taken together, these surrogate tests might eliminate about 60% of cases of post-transfusion NANB: a prediction that was eventually proven to be true. While the association of ALT with hepatitis infectivity was not unexpected, the relationship between anti-HBc and NANB was less easy to grasp. In large part, it was attributed to the similar epidemiology of the two agents. In retrospect, it was probably due to only those presenting blood donors who had a history (perhaps long past) of injecting drug use. Some blood centers implemented ALT screening of donors in the early 1980s, prior to the recognition of anti-HBc as a surrogate marker for NANB. Further progress in this area was temporarily set aside as a result of the appearance of the epidemic of HIV/AIDS. Table 3 outlines the improvements in the risk of transfusion-transmitted hepatitis over the years.

Table 3. Per-unit risk estimates for transfusion-transmitted HIV, United States

Year	Risk per unit	Notes	Reference
1988	1:40,000	Estimate based on assumed incidence	[38]
1989	1:153,000	Improved from Ward (10)	[39]
1991	1:160,000	Culture of seronegative donations	[40]
1992	1:60,000	Follow-up of transfused patients	[41]
1992	1:225,000	Window period plus incidence	[42]
1996	1:450,000	Window period plus incidence	[43]
1996	1:493,000	Window period plus incidence	[28]
1996	1:676,000	Impact of adding HIV p24 antigen test	[28]
2000	1:1,100,000	Impact of adding pooled NAT	*

* S.L. Stramer PhD, personal communication, May 2000.

It is of interest to note that, during the time of initial discussion about the implementation of ALT testing as a surrogate for NANB, blood bankers in particular questioned many facets of the issue, in a loose public forum. Concern was expressed that there were no controlled studies to establish the efficacy of the test. A subsequent study, performed in Canada, clearly did show that the approach would have been efficacious. Cost-benefit evaluations were performed, although they were rather inconclusive as it was hard to define the resource usage associated with NANB [14]. Many concluded that NANB was not a particularly severe disease. Blood collectors questioned the impact of a 1 to 2% deferral rate on the blood supply. This was an instance when individual blood systems or centers made their own decisions. Subsequent to the emergence of the AIDS epidemic, however, there was little hesitation to implement both ALT and anti-HBc as surrogates for NANB. Not only had the climate changed, but thought leaders had come to the conclusion that NANB was not a benign disease and encouraged intervention. Nevertheless, as will be noted below, there did continue to be some independence of thought and action in the early days of AIDS.

HIV/AIDS: days of turmoil

AIDS emerged as a completely new and unfamiliar disease, affecting a number of clearly defined "risk groups", among which were hemophilia patients receiving clotting factors made from pooled plasma. The primary epidemic emerged among men having sex with men and among injection drug users. Donald Francis, of the Centers for Disease Control and Prevention (CDC), must be credited with the recognition that this strange disease had characteristics consistent with an infectious etiology and further, that the agent was likely to be epidemiologically similar to HBV. He provided early warning to blood collectors, suggesting that they be alert to the disease and ready to take appropriate countermeasures. It was initially unclear what these measures should be, in the absence of any clear evidence of infectious etiology. A number of AIDS cases were eventually identified among individuals with blood transfusion as their only risk factor and in some of these cases, an implicated donor was subsequently found to have the disease [15,16]. Blood agencies, encouraged by the FDA, implemented measures to educate potential donors with risk factors and to encourage them not to give blood. Retrospective studies by Michael Busch showed how remarkably effective these measures were, at least in San Francisco, where the risk of transfusion transmitted AIDS dropped tenfold, from 1.2 per hundred blood units to less than 0.2%, prior to the availability of any test [17].

Another measure that was discussed was the use of anti-HBc as a surrogate marker. It had been shown that most individuals with AIDS, and many judged to be at high risk, were positive for anti-HBc. In this instance, this finding did emphasize a parallel epidemiology for the two agents. This approach was widely discussed, but only a small number of blood collection agencies adopted it. Much of this discussion was taking place at a time (May 1984) when Gallo and Montagnier had announced the identification of the putative etiologic agent of AIDS [18,19]. Also, Margaret Heckler, then Secretary of Health and Human Services, had stated that the US Government would manage the commercial development of a test within six months. (Licensure actually occurred in March of 1985). There were many social and ethical issues relating to the potential use of tests and there was also concern that the availability of tests in the blood bank environment would lead to test-seeking by those at risk. The development of so-called alternate test sites seemed to have been quite successful in minimizing this outcome.

Once ELISA tests for antibodies to HIV became available, they were rapidly and essentially uniformly implemented. Early data from the American Red Cross system showed that the frequency of reactive results was 0.038%, an indication of significant risk immediately prior to test implementation [20]. Also of concern was the finding that many of the seropositive donors did have established risk factors for AIDS. This observation led directly to a more intensive and detailed process of questioning blood donors. The FDA was heavily involved in developing the questions.

Table 4. Risk of transfusion transmitted hepatitis viruses, United States

Year	Agent	Risk	Notes	Reference
1968	PTH*	30%	Per patient, based on ALT elevation	[44]
1981	NANB†	11%	Per patient, based on ALT elevation	[10, 12]
1992	HCV	1:222	Per unit, before surrogate testing	[45]
1992	HCV	1:526	Per unit, addition of surrogate testing	[45]
1992	HCV	1:3,300	Per unit, addition of anti-HCV (1.0)	[45]
1995	HBV	1:250,000	Per unit, based on test sensitivity	[46]
1996	HBV	1:63,000	Per unit, window period plus incidence	[28]
1996	HCV	1:103,000	Per unit, window period plus incidence	[28]
2000	HCV	1:250,000	Per unit, addition of pooled NAT	‡

* PTH: Posttransfusion hepatitis, all cases, all causes

† NANB: Non-A, Non-B hepatitis

‡ S.L. Stramer, PhD: personal communication, May 2000

Overall, the AIDS epidemic is a global catastrophe and will continue to be for the foreseeable future, particularly where resources are limited. A component of the tragedy was the transmission of this disease to recipients of blood and blood components. Although such transmission has been almost entirely eliminated in the developed world, it is still a continuing threat in much of the developing world. There has been an almost global reevaluation of the response of the blood industry to AIDS and the outcomes have been largely critical and, in some cases, have led to criminal prosecution and/or major changes in the management of blood systems. Certainly, with today's knowledge in hand, the critiques are hard to counter. Yet the epidemic was entirely new and puzzling and the situation was by no means as clear at the time. Perhaps the most significant difficulty was the failure to recognize the unusual length of the incubation period for AIDS, and consequently, the size of the epidemic of infection that had already occurred, well before the appearance of any clinical cases. The appearance of AIDS was undoubtedly the second seminal event relating to blood safety. Table 4 outlines improvements in the risk of transfusion-transmitted HIV infection.

The impact of AIDS: a move towards "zero-risk"

As pointed out above, the advent of AIDS had a tremendous impact on attitudes about blood safety. Indeed, safety itself became the primary focus of decision making and there was relatively little hesitation to develop and implement additional screening measures designed to decrease risk. The first decision after the implementation of HIV antibody testing was to initiate surrogate testing for NANB in 1986-87. This was followed shortly by testing for HTLV-I in 1988.

This was probably the first test to be implemented in the United States prior to the recognition of a transfusion-transmitted case of the accompanying disease. Even so, such disease had been seen in other parts of the world. Also, it may not be widely appreciated that the decision was not data-free. Alan Williams and his colleagues performed a careful sero-epidemiologic study, showing that about 0.025% of US blood donors were positive for antibodies to HTLV. Risk factors were identified: they were primarily geographic for those donors whose reactivity was due to HTLV-I infection, and primarily drug-related for those infected with HTLV-II [21]. Subsequent lookback studies revealed that the viruses had been transmitted by transfusion of cellular products [22].

During this time, the FDA became much more active in driving blood safety issues. There was particular concern about the impact of a number of obvious gaps in testing capability. In particular, even though it was recognized to be very rare in the United States, the FDA required the use of tests for HIV-2, clearly stating a timeline for implementation, once licensed tests were available. This attitude has continued, as the Agency pressed for inclusion of specific HIV-1 group O antigens into US tests and subsequently, the inclusion of specific HTLV-II antigens into HTLV antibody tests (even though alternate approaches were shown to be efficacious). The FDA started to become much more vigilant about procedural aspects of blood collection, processing and distribution and continued to develop guidance and requirements relating to donor questioning.

Biotechnology makes its mark

The third seminal event was the cloning of a segment of the genome of the hepatitis C virus by Michael Houghton and his colleagues at Chiron, using virus grown in chimpanzees by Daniel Bradley, working at CDC [23,24]. This outcome was reported in 1989 and a serologic test became available in 1990. This was an heroic effort, involving the blind expression of presumed genomic fragments in bacteria and the examination of millions of clones for evidence of peptides that would react immunologically with convalescent serum from a case of NANB hepatitis. Once the key clone was found, the genome segment could be sequenced and used as a primary probe to walk the viral genome. The first (1.0) version of the anti-HCV test used only a single peptide from HCV as the capture reagent and was, in retrospect, neither particularly sensitive nor specific. Nevertheless, its use undoubtedly prevented the transmission of many thousands of cases of HCV infection. Within two years, a second version of the test became available, incorporating other recombinant HCV antigens. The current, 3.0 version uses an additional peptide, expressed from the NS-5 region and other antigens that have been modified to improve specificity. Although biotechnology had been used to some extent in the development of tests for other infection markers (e.g. for the production of recombinant or synthetic peptides as test kit components), HCV was the first instance in which the virus itself had been identified purely by nucleic acid-based technology.

It soon became apparent that the majority of cases of post-transfusion NANB were indeed caused by HCV and additionally, that once multi-antigen tests had been implemented, post-transfusion hepatitis declined to the extent that its incidence was no longer measurable by prospective studies. There were still a few unexplained cases of post-transfusion hepatitis, and the search for etiologic agents continues. Indeed, at least three putative hepatitis viruses have been reported in the past 5 years, but none can be definitively identified as a significant pathogen. In all cases, genomic techniques have been used; the principal connection with hepatitis has been that the isolation was from one or more patients with a diagnosis of hepatitis. The GBV-C and HGV agents have proven to be essentially identical and are flavi-like viruses, similar to HCV. The TT virus, in contrast, is a DNA virus, perhaps a circo virus, and SEN-V is also a DNA virus. All of these viruses are clearly transmissible by transfusion, and their nucleic acids can be found at surprisingly high frequency among healthy blood donors. But it does not appear to be possible to link any of these viruses unequivocally with post-transfusion disease. Despite the continuing anxiety about blood safety, it is of interest to note that there has been little impetus to develop or implement routine tests for any of these isolates. It is quite likely that modern technology will find many more such viruses in search of a disease. Indeed, these may be the smartest of all viruses, having dispensed with pathogenicity and existing quietly and peacefully within their host.

Window dressing: risk rehabilitated

A number of lines of evidence indicated that serologic testing, particularly for HIV and HCV, was imperfect. A few cases of HIV infection had been identified from HIV-antibody negative donations, some of which were positive for a soluble HIV antigen (p24). Additionally, studies of seroconverting individuals showed that p24 appeared before anti-HIV. A large study was performed in 1990 to assess whether implementation of p24 testing would have any significant impact on blood safety [25]. Around half a million routine donations were tested and none was found positive. This is hardly surprising, as the eventual implementation of p24 testing generated a yield of 1 antigen positive per five to nine million or more donations in the US. This study, along with other data, led to an open decision not to implement p24 antigen testing at that time, but the decision was reversed in 1995. Concern about residual HIV infection continued and two major lines of work were undertaken to assess the extent of this risk. The first was definition of the window period itself. Lookback studies showed that, up to 1990, HIV infection was transmitted by 20% of HIV-seronegative donations from individuals whose next donation was seropositive. Mathematical modeling indicated that the infectious window period for such donors was 45 days [26,42]. The other line of study was careful evaluation of serial samples taken at frequent intervals during seroconversion. Panels of such samples were developed from commercial plasma donors. Examination of these panels revealed that infection could be detected earlier in time as a result of using more sensitive tests for HIV antibodies, but also by use of HIV antigen tests and ultimately, by testing directly for viral RNA [27]. By combining these window period estimates with the incidence of new infection among routine donors, it was possible to estimate the residual risk of infection from donor blood. Further, it was possible to predict the impact of adding new tests as they decreased the length of the window period.

Similar data were developed for HTLV, HCV and HBV, although in these cases, the window period was defined essentially on the basis of elapsed time between exposure and appearance of serological markers. There is now clear data on the evolution of infection markers for the three major transfusion viruses. These window period estimates were used to estimate the overall risk of transfusion transmitted infections in the United States and were published in 1996 in a masterful study that has not yet been supplanted [28]. Although the residual risk estimates were largely comforting, they clearly were not zero, neither were they less than one in one million, which has been suggested as an "acceptable risk" in some other contexts. In 1994, David Kessler, then Commissioner of the FDA, called a public workshop and declared that even a single HIV transmission by transfusion was one too many. He encouraged the participants to develop and implement direct tests for viral nucleic acids for blood screening. At the time, this was considered to be an almost impossible objective that would not even be approached within a five-year time frame. Again, blood collectors were heard to say "we'll never be able to do that in the blood center". Yet, within five years, nucleic acid amplification testing for HIV and HCV was essentially uniformly in place in the US, albeit under IND and in pooled, rather than single samples. In the interim, it was recognized that, at least for HIV, Dr Kessler's objectives could be met in part, if tests for HIV p24 antigen were to be implemented. This was undertaken, but the yield was unexpectedly low.

GAT, NAT or GNAT?

Driven in part by Kessler's vision, in part by European initiatives designed to reduce the viral load in plasma for further manufacture, and in part by the availability of technology, US blood collectors, in collaboration with industry, developed and implemented programs for testing donations for HIV and HCV RNA. If the objective was to reduce transfusion-transmitted infection, then these programs have been successful. Within the Red Cross program, after one year of testing, 22 HCV positive and one HIV positive samples were identified, representing respective rates of 1 in 300,000 and 1 in 6.6 million. While these yields appear to be low, a recent analysis (Dodd et al, unpublished observations) shows that these findings, at least among repeat donors, are entirely consistent with estimated yields derived from current measures of incidence and estimates of RNA-positive window periods (Table 5). Another question is whether there is still an infectious window period during which RNA is not detectable, even if single samples are tested. Given today's pooled testing approach, and the relatively low initial levels of RNA in early HIV infection, it is certainly possible that a few cases of HIV-infectious donations may miss detection in pools. On the other hand, a provocative animal study is consistent with the concept that there may be no HIV infectivity before RNA is detectable [29]. Whether this is also true of HCV remains to be seen, and studies are currently in the design phase. Perhaps zero-risk can be achieved by testing alone.

Table 5. Yield of HIV and HCV RNA+, serology - donations, ARC, 1999-2000: Expected vs observed

Agent	FD: Observed ($n = 1.45 \times 10^6$)	RD: Observed ($n = 5.14 \times 10^6$)	RD: Expected*
HCV	11	11	12.6
HIV	0	1	1.2

* Expected numbers calculated from incidence rates in Table * and RNA window periods of 40 days for HCV, 5 days for HIV.

It is of some interest to speculate on the future of nucleic acid testing. Will there be a move to test for other agents? Certainly, there is continued interest in expanding the repertoire of testing of plasma for further manufacture, with measures already partly in place for HBV and the B19 parvo virus. It is unclear whether such measures will (or should) extend to single donor products. What is perhaps more important is that the availability of the nucleic acid testing platform implies a much more rapid track to the implementation of testing for new agents. It is clear that the technology of genomic detection and characterization of new agents is the method of choice. Indeed, HGV, TTV and SEN-V, like HCV, are known only through their genomes. It is surely much easier to develop primers and probes than to express antigens and raise antibodies.

Inactivation of pathogens

Over the past fifteen years, a great deal of attention has been paid to pathogen inactivation. Pooled plasma products are now essentially completely safe as a result of a variety of additive procedures and much progress has been made in the search for inactivation protocols for single donor products. Indeed, virally inactivated and quarantined (i.e. donor re-tested) frozen plasma has been available for several years. At least one approach for inactivation of viruses and bacteria in platelets has reached phase III clinical trials and a method for red cells is progressing along the same track.

The term inactivation seems to imply that infectivity will be eliminated from cellular components. In practice, this may occur, at least for the major transfusion-transmissible agents, but only because inactivation will be used in concert with highly effective testing. Inactivation is not an all-or-nothing phenomenon and there is always an aspect of dose-response and time-response that establishes the maximum capability of any process. In addition, it must be recognized that many viruses are relatively resistant to damage, while blood cells are not. As a consequence, inactivation procedures must achieve a delicate balance between the two objectives of removing infectivity and sparing cellular function. This is one of the major reasons favoring inactivation methods that are specific for nucleic acids, as the therapeutic efficacy of red cells and platelets is not dependent upon the presence or functionality of RNA or DNA. Nevertheless, review of available data suggests that inactivation procedures are probably unable to eliminate more than about 6-7 $\log_{10}$ of infectivity for target (or appropriate model) viruses. Consider however, that NAT testing (which will likely be required to have analytical sensitivity of 100 genome equivalents/mL) can identify window period donations with RNA levels greater than 1600 to 2400 geq/mL in pooled testing; non-window period donations should be detectable by serologic tests. Thus, assuming that one genome equivalent is equal to one infectious dose (an assumption that is probably far too sensitive), then an inactivation method would not have to deal with more than about 3×10^5 hepatitis C or human immunodeficiency viruses per 200 mL component. The levels of HBV DNA appear to be significantly lower than this in seronegative samples, and HTLV and CMV are present at low titer and are almost exclusively cell-associated. Data for S-59 (the psoralen derivative that is currently under evaluation for treatment of platelet concentrates), show that at least 10^4 to 10^5 colony forming units of bacteria are inactivated (30). It is likely that this approach will essentially eliminate bacterial risk, as the titer of bacterial contaminants is thought to be much lower that this when the components are manufactured.

The additional benefit of such inactivation procedures will be small and the costs will likely be appreciable. Whether the benefits will drive widespread adoption remains to be seen, and elsewhere in this volume, James AuBuchon discusses the dynamics of decision making in the context of blood safety. There seems to be a general opinion that the value of inactivation will lie in its ability to prevent transmission of new diseases via transfusion, yet there is no way to estimate the risk of the emergence of another blood-borne infectious agent. Further, it should be noted that the titers of viral agents in the blood can readily exceed the capabilities of inactivation methods that preserve blood cell function. Thus, the promise of inactivation may turn out to be hollow in the context of novel infections.

Whither (or wither) confirmatory testing?

Although screening tests for donors have impressively high sensitivity and specificity, they are used on a population with a remarkably low prevalence of infection. As a consequence, the positive predictive value of these tests is low. Confirmatory or supplemental testing is intended to improve the accuracy of the primary screening test result, in order to provide responsible and medically accurate information to the donor. Unfortunately, most of the tests used for this purpose are far from satisfactory, often yielding more "indeterminate" results than positive or negative ones [31]. The immunologic blocking technique used as a confirmatory procedure for HBsAg was generally accurate, except when used for samples with very low signal levels. Unfortunately, this approach cannot be used effectively for tests in which antibodies are the analyte. When the first anti-HIV test was described, an accompanying paper discussed the use of a western blot procedure to confirm the presence of antibodies [32]. As a result, this technique was drawn into the mainstream and became the standard for assessing donor samples with reactive EIA results. Western blot tests were eventually licensed by the FDA as a supplementary "more specific" test for HIV antibodies. This enshrined the approach and western blots are used for "confirmation" of HTLV and the somewhat similar strip immunoassay is used for

HCV. Because of the undue frequency of indeterminate outcomes, many completely health donors are presented with an essentially incomprehensible message about their status. Licensure of these blot procedures has inhibited the adoption of alternate approaches and the situation is compounded by a proposed regulation to require the use of a licensed confirmatory test for all EIA reactive findings. It would be much better to step back from the blot and consider the use of an objective procedure (such as NAT) to confirm EIA reactivity.

Are we marching backwards into the future?

An impressive edifice of blood safety measures has been constructed over the last 60 years, with most of the action taking place in the past 15 years. We not only have tests of exquisite sensitivity and specificity, but we also have detailed knowledge about the pathology and epidemiology of donor infection. We continue to search for new ways to assess and reduce risk and we have expanded our horizons to cover exotic and imported infections. We have a system of ever more detailed, overlapping measures to support and maintain blood safety. We have decision systems that now extend to implementing measures that are designed to reduce risks that are openly defined as "theoretical". We continue to expand the length and intensity of our donor questionnaire (or, as Merlyn Sayers called it: donor interrogation). All of these measures are tied together, quite properly, by documentation, review and quality systems. But, it is evident that every new measure has been added to those that already existed. Many would like to think that this has resulted in an impenetrable and solid structure – a massive series of brick walls, perhaps. But there is also concern that the edifice is too complex and costly and that it may even be counterproductive. Interestingly, even the very conservative "Precautionary Principle", which is much in vogue as a decision tool in Europe, eschews the concepts of zero risk and disproportionate response [33].

There have been some attempts to reevaluate components of the system, but in truth, little has been achieved. An excellent Consensus Development Conference reviewed the continued value of a number of tests in 1995 [34]. It was concluded that, in the presence of effective tests for antibodies to HCV, there was little value in continuing to test for elevated ALT levels. ALT testing was never required or recommended by the FDA and a number of blood establishments did stop testing. Many others continued, as manufacturers of pooled plasma products still require that plasma for further manufacture be tested for elevated ALT. As an aside, it is of interest to note that donations that are HCV RNA-positive, antibody negative, frequently have elevated ALT levels (8 of 22 RNA positive, anti-HCV negative donations in the Red Cross system, for example). The conference also concluded that neither anti-HBc nor syphilis testing had any significant value as a surrogate for other infections. Yet the first was thought to have some value (albeit small) in reducing transfusion-transmitted HBV, and the value of syphilis testing could not be assessed. Thus, it was recommended that, in the absence of any contrary evidence, testing should continue.

Within the year 1999, the FDA indicated, in a proposed set of regulations for donor testing, that it would be willing to review data presented in support of elimination of testing for syphilis. Preliminary data on about 100 donor samples that were selected on the basis of a positive test result for syphilis indicated that none of them had any evidence of the presence of *Treponema pallidum* genomic sequences [35]. A much larger study with negative findings would be necessary to support any change in regulatory position.

It is widely anticipated that it will be possible to demonstrate that all donor samples that are truly positive for HIV-1 p24 antigen will also be positive by NAT. Thus, it may be possible to eliminate the p24 antigen test once a NAT procedure is licensed by the FDA. This possibility was anticipated when the FDA recommended the implementation of p24 testing as an interim measure, pending the availability of more sensitive tests.

There have also been discussions about the nature and value of at least some donor questions. Unfortunately, to date, there has been no significant reduction in the intensity or number of required questions. Indeed, there have been substantial increases in the number of questions. In particular, complex questions have been required to reduce the theoretical risk of transmission of CJD or variant CJD by transfusion: the latter measure was actually anticipated to eliminate more than 2% of current donors in the US. Even more complex questions have been proposed in anticipation that xeno-transplantation might introduce viruses of animal origin into the blood supply. In spite of clear evidence that donors fail to respond correctly to risk questions about 2% of the time, there is no program to validate any of existing or proposed questions for understanding. When studies have been performed to assess the extent to which questions are understood, the results suggest that the questions may fail to achieve their anticipated purpose.

Perhaps an even more interesting topic is the extent to which donor questioning has any value in reducing the risk of infection, particularly when there are effective tests in place. Limited data, based upon incidence of infection among previously deferred donors, suggest, but by no means prove, that risk questioning may have little impact upon those who actually present to donate. On the other hand, it is quite possible that at-risk individuals never come to the blood center because they are aware that questions will be asked. In some cases, of course, questioning may be the barely strategy. For example, a history of travel or residence in a malarious area seems to be quite effective in controlling transfusion malaria in the US. There are approximately 1,000 cases of imported malaria each year in the US, yet only 2-3 cases of transfusion malaria [36]. Presumably, the number would be ten- to twenty-fold higher if those incubating transfusion malaria donated at the 5% rate seen in the general population. On the other hand, the questions about travel, while sensitive, are clearly not at all specific. Consequently, at least in parts of Europe, there is a strategy that involves testing donors who report malaria risk and accepting those with negative results. The concept of examining existing procedures for obsolescence is important and creditable. But it is difficult to design ethically acceptable studies that can provide reassurance that removing a measure will not affect safety. Perhaps radical thinking is required and we should ask whether we do have to keep building on everything that went before, or whether we could reevaluate today's conditions and establish a new, but equally safe structure? In other words, suppose that we had all of today's knowledge, but could forget the history of blood safety, then what kind of a system would we construct to assure patient safety? This is a challenging question, and one that I would not attempt to answer, but it would be good to stimulate new thinking in this critical area.

Comment

Countless lives have been saved by blood transfusion. In the early days, the benefits of transfusion were clearly seen to outweigh the disadvantages. Yet over the past thirty years, it seems that the perception has been inverted and more and more effort has been devoted to the ever-decreasing risk of infection. This has led to a continuously increasing battery of blood safety measures. Although this has given us a blood supply that presents little direct risk to the patient, the complexity and cost of the processes may be reaching a point that is counterproductive. Further, the concept that society will pay any cost for blood safety has been challenged by the less-than enthusiastic adoption of measures such as virally-inactivated frozen plasma, universally leukocyte reduced components and even NAT. It is possible that some long-standing safety measures have been superseded by improved technologies or additional procedures. Responsible assessment of the value of each component of the blood safety complex should be conducted, with a view to eliminating the unnecessary and worthless without compromising the overall safety of the blood supply. Finally, we should ponder the inequities of putting so much in the way of resources into the safety of our own blood supply, when the real problem still lies in the developing world.

References

1. Barker LF. In: Dodd RY, Barker LF, eds. Infection, Immunity, and Blood Transfusion. New York: Alan R. Liss; 1985;Introduction. p. xix-xxv.
2. Allen JG. The epidemiology of posttransfusion hepatitis. Basic blood and plasma tabulations. Stanford: Commonwealth Fund; 1972. pp. 1-335
3. Krugman S, Giles JP, Hammond J. Infectious hepatitis. Evidence for two distinctive clinical, epidemiological, and immunological types of infection. JAMA 1967;200:365-73.
4. Tegtmeier GE, Parks LH, Blosser JK, et al. Hepatitis markers in blood donors with a history of hepatitis or jaundice. [Abstract] Transfusion 1991;31, Supplement:64S.
5. Blumberg BS, Alter HJ, Visnich S. A 'new' antigen in leukemia sera. JAMA 1965;191:541-46.
6. Blumberg BS, Gerstley BJS, Hungerford DA, London WT, Sutnick AI. A serum antigen (Australia antigen) in Down's syndrome, leukemia and hepatitis. Ann Intern Med 1967;66:924.
7. Gocke DJ, Greenberg HB, Kavey NB. Correlation of Australia antigen with posttransfusion hepatitis. JAMA 1970;212:877-79.

8. Ling CM, Overby LR. Prevalence of hepatitis B virus antigen as revealed by direct radioimmune assay with 125-I-antibody. J Immunol 1972;109:834-41.
9. Feinstone SM, Kapikian AZ, Purcell RH, Alter HJ, Holland PV. Transfusion-associated hepatitis not due to viral hepatitis type A or B. N Engl J Med 1975;292:767-70.
10. Alter HJ, Purcell RH, Holland PV, Alling DW, Koziol DE. Donor transaminase and recipient hepatitis. Impact on blood transfusion services. JAMA 1981;246:630-34.
11. Koziol DE, Holland PV, Alling DW, et al. Antibody to Hepatitis B core antigen as a paradoxical marker for non-A, non-B hepatitis agents in donated blood. Ann Intern Med. 1986;104:488-95.
12. Aach RD, Szmuness W, Mosley JW, et al. Serum alanine aminotransferase of donors in relation to the risk of non-A, non-B hepatitis in recipients. The Transfusion-Transmitted Viruses Study. N Engl J Med 1981;304:989-94.
13. Stevens CE, Aach RD, Hollinger FB, et al. Hepatitis B virus antibody in blood donors and the occurrence of Non-A, non-B hepatitis in transfusion recipients. An analysis of the Transmission-Transmitted Viruses Study. Ann Intern Med. 1984;101:733-38.
14. Hornbrook MC, Dodd RY, Jacobs P, Friedman LI, Sherman KE. Reducing the incidence of non-A, non-B post-transfusion hepatitis by testing donor blood for alanine aminotransferase. Economic considerations. New Engl J Med 1982;307:1315-21.
15. Curran JW, Lawrence DN, Jaffe H, et al. Acquired immunodeficiency syndrome (AIDS) associated with transfusions. N Engl J Med 1984;310:69-75.
16. Peterman TA, Jaffe HW, Feorino PM, et al. Transfusion-associated acquired immunodeficiency syndrome in the United States. JAMA 1985;254:2913-17.
17. Busch MP, Young MJ, Samson SM, Mosley JW, Ward JW, Perkins HA, Transfusion Safety Study Group. Risk of human immunodeficiency virus (HIV) transmission by blood transfusions before the implementation of HIV-1 antibody screening. Transfusion 1991;31:4-11.
18. Gallo RC, Salahuddin SZ, Popovic M, et al. Frequent detection and isolation of cytopathic retroviruses (HTLV-III) from patients with AIDS and at risk for AIDS. Science 1984;224:500-03.
19. Barre-Sinoussi F, Chermann J-C, Rey F, et al. Isolation of a T-lymphotropic retrovirus from a patient at risk for acquired immune deficiency syndrome (AIDS). Science 1983;220:868-71.
20. Schorr JB, Berkowitz A, Cumming PD, Katz AJ, Sandler SG. Prevalence of HTLV-III antibody in American blood donors. N Engl J Med 1985;313:384-85.
21. Williams AE, Fang CT, Slamon DJ, et al. Seroprevalence and epidemiological correlates of HTLV-1 infection in U.S. blood donors. Science 1988; 240:643-46.
22. Sullivan MT, Williams AE, Fang CT, et al. Transmission of human T-lymphotropic virus types I and II by blood transfusion: A retrospective study of recipients of blood components (1983 through 1988). Arch Intern Med. 1991;151:2043-48.

23. Choo Q-L, Kuo G, Weiner AJ, Overby LR, Bradley DW, Houghton M. Isolation of a cDNA clone derived from a blood borne non-A, non-B viral hepatitis genome. Science 1989;244:359-62.
24. Kuo G, Choo Q-L, Alter HJ, Gitnick GL, et al. An assay for circulating antibodies to a major etiologic virus of human non-A, non-B hepatitis. Science 1989;244:362-64.
25. Alter HJ, Epstein JS, Swenson SG, et al. Prevalence of human immunodeficiency virus type 1 p24 antigen in U.S. blood donors--An assessment of the efficacy of testing in donor screening. N Engl J Med. 1990;323:1312-17.
26. Petersen LR, Satten G, Dodd RY, et al. Current estimates of the infectious window period and risk of HIV infection from seronegative blood donations. [Abstract] Program and Abstracts: Fifth National Forum on AIDS, Hepatitis, and Other Blood-Borne Diseases 1992;37.
27. Busch MP, Lee LLL, Satten GA, Henrard DR, et al. Time course of detection of viral and serologic markers preceding human immunodeficiency virus type 1 seroconversion: Implications for screening of blood and tissue donors. Transfusion 1995;35:91-97.
28. Schreiber GB, Busch MP, Kleinman SH, Korelitz JJ. The risk of transfusion-transmitted viral infections. N Engl J .Med. 1996;334:1685-90.
29. Murthy KK, Henrard DR, Eichberg JW, Cobb KE, Busch MP, Allain JP, Alter HJ. Redefining the HIV-infectious window period in the chimpanzee model: evidence to suggest that viral nucleic acid testing can prevent blood-borne transmission. Transfusion 1999;39:688-93.
30. Corash L. Virus inactivation in cellular components. Vox Sang. 1996;70 (Suppl. 3):9-16.
31. Dodd RY, Stramer SL. Indeterminate results in blood donor testing: What you don't know can hurt you. Transfus Med Rev 2000;14:151-60.
32. Sarngadharan MG, Popovic M, Bruch L, Schupbach J, Gallo RC. Antibodies reactive with human T-lymphotropic retroviruses (HTLV-III) in the serum of patients with AIDS. Science 1984;224:506-08.
33. Foster KR, Vecchia P, Repacholi MH. Risk management. Science and the precautionary principle. Science 2000;288:979-81.
34. Desforges JF, Athari F, Cooper ES, et al. Infectious disease testing for blood transfusions. JAMA 1995;274:1374-79.
35. Orton SL, ARCNET Program, Liu H, et al. Prevalence of circulating T. pallidum in STS+/FTA-ABS+ blood donors. [Abstract] Transfusion 2000; 39:(S)2S.
36. Nahlen BL, Lobel HO, Cannon SE, Campbell CC. Reassessment of blood donor selection criteria for United States travellers to malarious areas. Transfusion 1991;31:798-804.
37. Dodd RY, Stramer SL, Aberle-Grasse J, Notari E. Risk of hepatitis and retroviral infections among blood donors and introduction of nucleic acid testing (NAT). Dev Biol Stand 2000;102:19-27.
38. Ward JW, Holmberg SD, Allen JR, et al. Transmission of human immunodeficiency virus (HIV) by blood transfusions screened as negative for HIV antibody. N.Engl J Med. 1988;318:473-78.

39. Cumming PD, Wallace EL, Schorr JB, Dodd RY. Exposure of patients to human immunodeficiency virus through the transfusion of blood components that test antibody-negative. N Engl J Med. 1989;321:941-46.
40. Busch MP, Eble BE, Khayam-Bashi H, et al. Evaluation of screened blood donations for human immunodeficiency virus type 1 infection by culture and DNA amplification of pooled cells. N Engl J Med. 1991;325:1-5.
41. Nelson KE, Donahue JG, Muñoz A, et al. Transmission of retroviruses from seronegative donors by transfusion during cardiac surgery. A multicenter study of HIV-1 and HTLV-I/II infections. Ann Intern Med. 1992;117:554-59.
42. Petersen LR, Satten GA, Dodd R, et al. HIV Seroconversion Study Group. Duration of time from onset of human immunodeficiency virus type 1 infectiousness to development of detectable antibody. Transfusion 1994;34: 283-89.
43. Lackritz EM, Satten GA, Aberle-Grasse J et al. Estimated risk of transmission of the human immunodeficiency virus by screened blood in the United States. N Engl J Med. 1995;333:1721-25.
44. Alter HJ. You'll wonder where the yellow went: A 15-year retrospective of posttransfusion hepatitis. In: Moore SB, editor. Transfusion-Transmitted Viral Diseases. Arlington, VA: AABB; 1987; 4:p. 53-86.
45. Donahue JG, Muñoz A, Ness PM, et al. The declining risk of post-transfusion hepatitis C virus infection. N Engl J Med. 1992;327:369-73.
46. Alter, MJ Residual risk of transfusion-associated hepatitis. Bethesda, MD: National Institutes of Health; NIH Consensus Development Conference on Infectious Disease Testing for Blood Transfusions. 1995; 23.

QUALITY MANAGEMENT FOR BLOOD TRANSFUSION SERVICES[1]

Gaby Vercauteren[2]

The safety and adequacy of blood and blood products still cannot be ensured in many WHO Member States. A priority strategic area is to adopt the principles of *quality management* in all areas of the blood transfusion services in order to ensure good organisation, management, donation from safe blood donors, testing of all donated blood for HIV and other transfusion transmissible infections and, on a consistent basis, provide for quality component production and appropriate clinical use of blood.

WHO identified that urgent action needed to be devoted to developing a quality management project for blood transfusion services in all regions. This activity involves a strong training and information component covering the different aspects of quality assurance as well as the establishment of regional external quality assessment schemes for transfusion transmissible infections and for blood group serology.

The objectives of the quality management project for blood transfusion services are to:

- Assist Member States to improve blood safety and prevent HIV, HCV and HBV transmission, by identifying and implementing key strategies.
- Improve the capacity, skills and knowledge of Member States in all regions in the area of blood and blood product safety.
- Establish regional external quality assessment schemes (EQAS) for blood group serology and transfusion transmissible infections.
- Develop regional and interregional networks.

The establishment of one or more regional training centres for quality management for blood transfusion services will build regional as well as national capacity. The approach involves the provision of training covering all aspects of blood transfusion management and offering participation in regional quality assessment schemes. Progress made by the participating blood transfusion services will be monitored and evaluated at regular time intervals. Hence a cycle of continuous improvement through training and assessment will have been created. This integrated approach has the potential to improve blood safety in the Region in a relatively short time span.

---

1. Eds: No manuscript available.
2. WHO Department of Blood Safety and Clinical Technology, Geneva, CH.

THE VALUE OF DONOR SELECTION FOR BLOOD SAFETY[1]

Cees L. van der Poel[2]

Any chain is as strong as its weakest link. This is a Dutch saying, and readily applicable to the blood transfusion chain. Not strictly Dutch though is our stubborn unwillingness to pay blood donors for their donations. Why? Is it our well known strive for cost-containment? Not sure. Voluntary non-remunerated donation is the basis for a safe blood transfusion policy. This is the single most powerful achievement of transfusion safety since the nineteen-seventies. However as with any powerful kingdom, its sovereignty is readily down-played. Not because of new medical or scientific insights, but more down to earth by financial interests. The king is not dead yet however.

The – safety of – the blood transfusion chain involves selection of donors, collection of blood, testing procedures, production processes, storage and transport, proper selection of patients who need to be transfused, and the selection of the proper blood products they are to receive. Quality Assurance programmes encompass the processes of the whole transfusion chain and hemovigilance programmes include active surveillance of adverse events in the whole chain. But donor selection is the start of it all.

During the last decades, new blood borne agents have been discovered, and new tests have been implied. On precisely all of these occasions, paid blood donors have proven to be of higher risk than non-remunerated donors. It may be reasoned that just the very introduction of these new tests will further eliminate the difference in risk among these donor populations. This is certainly true for the known tests and the known viruses. But since history has repeatedly taught us this lesson at the introduction of every new test for a newly discovered agent, are we to sit and wait for a new virus to come and teach us again? Paid donors simply pose higher risks of blood borne infections than non-remunerated ones. Alternative safety measures may be taken by industries to compensate for a higher risk once this is recognised. Examples are NAT testing, new categorisation of donors, insertion of an on-hold period for source plasma to anticipate inadvertent donations, additional inactivation procedures etc. But when these very same measures become state of the art and are shared by most transfusion systems, the discussion is back to its source: the blood donor.

The safety of blood donors also depends on the degree to which donors understand the content and importance of the information they receive at the donor

1. Eds: manuscript not received.
2. Sanquin Blood Supply Foundation, Amsterdam, NL.

centres. The more they become educated in transfusion matters, the more they are able to properly understand their own responsibilities. Such effects have been indirectly measured by using adapted screening assays to detect sero-conversions in new donors, where it was found that new donors have a higher incidence of infections such as HIV.

A sufficient blood supply may be an issue to affect donor selection. The benefits of transfusion have to be weighed against its possible side-effects. The lack of transfusion blood may be considered a risk as well. In developing countries it is accepted, that some safety measures are not employed, not only because of the costs but also because the lack of sufficient donors. In some highly industrialised countries, with formerly a sufficient blood supplies, presently the accumulation of safety measures has added to shortages in the blood supply. In these countries some safety measures are now reconsidered. Some measures may have questionable effects on the blood safety. Interestingly, public awareness issues and not so much scientific arguments are leading policies into readily deferring large percentages of well-educated donors, taking risks by replacing them with new donors. This in a time that shortages are claimed as an excuse to pay donors, forcing the very same policy makers to abandon important safety measures that have proven to be of value, and install new ones that are not.

BLOOD DONATION; A RISK FOR PRENATAL DEVELOPMENTAL TOXICITY?

P.W.J. Peters[1]

Introduction

Most prescribers and users of drugs are familiar with the cautions on drug use during the first trimester of pregnancy. These warnings were introduced after the thalidomide disaster in the early 1960s. However, limiting the exercise of caution to the first 3 months of pregnancy is both short sighted and effectively impossible. First, because chemicals can affect any stage of pre- or postnatal development, and second, because when a woman first learns that she is pregnant, the process of organogenesis has already long since begun, for example, the neural walls are closed. In the case of blood donations there exists a possibility that medicinal products, prescribed to donors or used by them as "over the counter" drugs can become available in the recipients of blood donations. Hence, it is interesting not only to focus on blood donation as such but also to discuss here in general the developmental toxicity of biologically active substances and especially medicinal products. Blood donation is in this context then a special route of exposure. This text will present the current state of knowledge about the (un)safety of the use of medicinal products, including those that might be presented by blood donation in pregnancy. One must realise that to my knowledge there exists no literature or other data showing such hazard and risk. However, biological active substances might be transferred by blood donation into recipients. Hence, it will be important to understand the main issues in the field of reproductive and developmental toxicology. A recent guide about the safety of use of drugs during pregnancy and lactation is edited by Schaefer [1].

Development and health

During pregnancy there is the need to avoid harmful medicinal products, either prescribed, or taken as over-the-counter drugs, or drugs of abuse, including cigarettes and alcohol, as well as occupational and environmental exposure to potentially harmful chemicals [2]. Obviously sufficient and well-balanced nutrition is also essential [3]. When such primary preventive measures are neglected complications of pregnancy and developmental disorders can result. Further-

1. Professor of Teratology, University Medical Centre Utrecht, Utrecht, NL Chief Inspector Food, Inspectorate for Health Protection and Veterinary Public Health, 's-Gravenhage, NL.

more, nutritional deficiencies and toxic effects during prenatal life predispose the future adult to some diseases, such as metabolic imbalances, diabetes and cardiovascular illnesses, as demonstrated by Barker [4] based upon epidemiological and experimental data.

Reproductive stages

The different stages of reproduction are in fact highlights of a continuum

Primordial germ cells are present in the embryo at about one month after the first day of the last menstruation (figure 1). They subsequently differentiate into oogonia and oocytes or into spermatogonia. The oocytes in postnatal life are at an arrested stage of the meiotic division. This division is restarted much later after birth, shortly before ovulation and is finalised after fertilisation with the expulsion of the polar bodies. Thus, all female germ cells develop prenatally and no germ cells are formed after birth; moreover, during female life span approximately 400 oocytes undergo ovulation. All these facts make it possible to state that an 8-week pregnant mother of an unborn female is already a half grandmother!

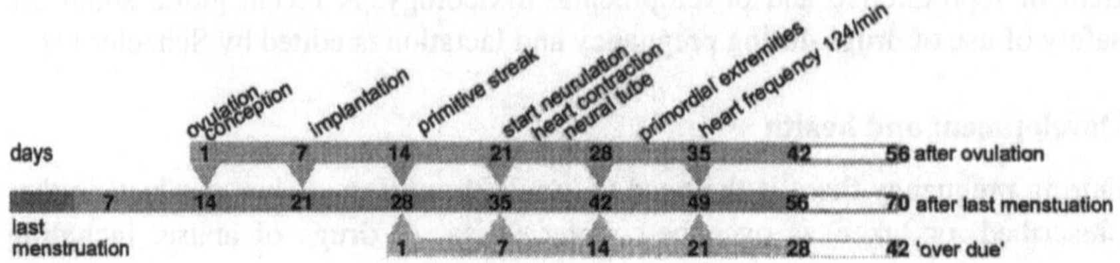

Figure 1.Timetable of early human development.

The embryonal spermatogenic epithelium, on the contrary, divides slowly by repeated mitoses; these cells do not differentiate into spermatocytes and do not undergo meiosis in the prenatal period. The onset of meiosis in the male begins at puberty. Spermatogenesis continues throughout (reproductive) life.

After fertilisation of the oocyte by one of the spermatozoa in the oviduct there is the stage of cell divisions and transport of the blastocyst into the endocrine-prepared uterine cavity. After implantation the bilaminar stage is formed and embryogenesis starts. The next 7 weeks are a period of finely balanced cellular events, including proliferation, migration, association, differentiation, and programmed cell death precisely arranged to produce tissues and organs from the genetic information, present in each conceptus. During this period of organogenesis rapid cell multiplication is the rule. Complex processes of cell migration, pattern formation and the penetration of one cell group by another, characterise the later stages.

Final morphological and functional development occurs at different times during foetogenesis and is mostly only completed after birth. Postnatal adaptation characterises the passage from intra- into extra-uterine life with tremendous changes in, for example, circulatory and respiratory physiology.

Reproductive and developmental toxicology

Reproductive toxicology is the subject area dealing with the causes, mechanisms, effects and prevention of disturbances throughout the entire reproductive cycle, including fertility induced by chemicals. Teratology (derived from the Greek word teras: wonder, divine intervention) is the science concerned with birth defects of a structural nature.

Reproductive toxicity represents harmful effects by agents on the progeny and/or impairment of male and female reproductive functions. Developmental toxicity involves any adverse effect induced prior to attainment of adult life. It includes effects induced or manifested in the embryonic or foetal period and those induced or manifested postnatally. Embryo/foetotoxicity involves any toxic effect on the conceptus resulting from prenatal exposure, including structural and functional abnormalities of postnatal manifestations of such effects. Teratogenicity is a manifestation of developmental toxicity, representing a particular case of embryo/foetotoxicity, by the induction or the increase of the frequency of structural disorders in the progeny.

The rediscovery of Mendel's laws, and the knowledge that some congenital abnormalities were passed on from parents to children, led to attempts to explain abnormalities in children on the basis of genetic theory. However, Hale [5] noticed that piglets born to sows fed a vitamin A-deficient diet were born without eyes. His conclusion was that a nutritional deficiency leads to a marked disturbance of the internal factors that control the mechanism of eye development. During a rubella epidemic in 1941, the Australian ophthalmologist Gregg [6] observed that embryos, which had been exposed to the rubella virus often displayed abnormalities, such as cataracts, cardiac defects, deafness, and mental retardation. Soon after this it was discovered that the protozoon toxoplasma, a unicellular parasite, could induce abnormalities in the unborn. These observations proved undeniably that the placenta is not an absolute barrier against external influences.

Furthermore, in the early 1960s, maternal exposure to the mild sedative thalidomide appeared to be causing characteristic reduction deformities of the limbs ranging from hypoplasia of 1 or more digits to total absence of all limbs. An example of the thalidomide embryopathy is phocomelia: the structures of the hand and feet may be reduced to a single small digit or may appear virtually normal but protrude directly from the trunk, like the flippers of a seal. This discovery by Lenz [7] led to a world wide interest in clinical teratology.

An essential aim of public health is prevention. Primary prevention of developmental disorders can be defined as the use of methods to prevent the origin of a developmental disorder. This is in contrast to secondary prevention of developmental disorders, which means the prevention of the birth of a child with a developmental defect, usually by abortion.

The approach for primary prevention of birth defects is most successful when a medicinal product prevents the initiation of a disorder, for example rubella vaccination, or by correction of an aberrant lifestyle such as alcohol abuse. Moreover, primary prevention of developmental disorders can be achieved when a chemical substance is identified as a reproductive toxicant and is either not approved for marketing, or approved with specific pregnancy labelling, restricted in use, or removed from the market.

When thalidomide was recognised as the causal factor of phocomelia, removal of the drug from the market resulted in the disappearance of the embryopathy. This event was also accompanied by a transient drastic avoidance of general drug intake by pregnant women.

Healthcare professionals and pregnant women need to develop a more critical attitude to the use of medicinal products and exposure to chemicals not only during pregnancy but also before pregnancy, or even better, during the entire fertile period. Such a critical attitude could result in avoiding many unnecessary and unknown risks.

These remarks imply that health professionals, couples planning to have children, or pregnant women need to be informed about drugs proven to be safe, and about the risks of wanted or unwanted exposures to chemicals, including through blood donation.

Basic principles of drug-induced reproductive and developmental toxicology

Medicinal products that have the capacity to induce reproductive toxicity can be identified to some extent before being used or launched into the market by adapting the outcome of laboratory animal experiments. The final conclusions about (un)safety can only be awaited through epidemiological studies after the product has been some time on the market (post-launching surveillance). The determination of whether a given medicinal product has the potentiality or capability to induce developmental disorders is essentially governed by four established fundamental principles [8]. It can be stated that an embryo- and foetotoxic response depends upon the exposure to:

- A specific substance in a particular dose;
- A genetically susceptible species;

- A conceptus in a susceptible stage of development; and
- The mode of action of reproductive toxic drugs.

Principle 1: as in other toxicological evaluations, reproductive toxicity is governed by dose-effect relationships; the curve, however, is generally quite steep. The dose-response is of the utmost importance in determining if there is a true effect. Moreover, nearly every reproductive toxic drug that has been realistically tested or was clinically positive has been shown to have a 'no-effect' level. Another aspect worth mentioning here is the sometimes highly specific nature of the substance. For instance, thalidomide is a clear-cut teratogen in the human and specific species in contrast to its analogs that were never proven to be developmental toxicants. Moreover, not only is the daily dose of importance to result in a potential embryo/foetotoxic concentration of the drug, but also the route of exposure. This is obviously of importance when dealing with blood donations.

Principle 2: not all mammalian species are equally susceptible or sensitive to the reproductive toxic influence of a given chemical. Inter- and intraspecies variability may be manifested in several ways: a drug that acts in one species may have little or no effects in others; a reproductive toxicant may produce similar defects in various species, but these defects will vary in frequency. A substance may induce certain developmental disorders in one species that are entirely different from those induced in other. The explanation is that there are genetic differences that influence the teratogenic response. This may be further modified by environmental factors.

Principle 3: there exists a sensitive period for different effects, i.e. the developmental phase during which originating, proliferating and differentiating cells and organs become susceptible to a given drug. This period may not be related to critical morphogenetic periods, but may, for example, be related to the appearance of specific receptors. This explains how at an early period of development, dysmorphology is induced by a substance which, at the opposite end of the timetable of development, induces functional disorders such as those of the central nervous system.

Principle 4: the mode of action of reproductive toxic drugs. The pathogenesis and the final effects of developmental toxicity can be studied rather well. Knowledge about the early onset or the mechanism of this process of interference of agents with development is practically absent. Mechanistic information is, however, essential to understand how chemicals can disturb development and is a critical component of risk evaluation. To improve the understanding of the mode of action of toxicants, including early repair mechanisms, critical molecular targets of components of developmental processes should be identified. The signalling pathways that operate in the development of the organs of model animals, such as the fruit fly, roundworm and zebra fish, also operate in the development of mammalian organs; therefore the effects of medicinal products on fundamental processes such as signalling can be detected. Because the same signalling pathways operating in the various kinds of organ development in mammals are partially known and will be soon better known, a chemical's toxicological impact on these pathways can be predicted on the basis of the results in non-mammalian organisms and tested in mammals [9].

Effects and manifestations

A wide variety of responses characterises developmental toxicity. Infertility, chromosomal and genetic disorders, spontaneous abortion, intrauterine death, prematurity, low birth weight, birth defects and functional disorders are effects of such drug interference with developmental and reproductive processes. The manifestation of a developmental or reproductive toxicant can either be seen immediately after exposure or will be expressed at a much later date. Interfering with male or female germ cell development might result in infertility, decreased sperm activity and/or libido and impaired gametogenesis. Effects on the pre-implantation stage will cause early embryonic death, extrauterine implantation or delayed transport of the fertilised zygote.

A critical phase for the induction of structural malformations usually occurs during the period of organogenesis. In humans, this critical period extends from about 20-70 days after the first day of the last menstruation period, or from one week before the missed menstruation until the woman is 44 days 'overdue'. It may be unwise to rely absolutely on this time period. With physical agents such as X-rays used in laboratory animals, exposure can be limited exactly to a period of minutes to discover the exact sensitive period for inducing a specific disorder. However, in drugs or biological active substances such as in blood products we are not at all sure about the time courses of absorption, metabolism and excretion. In addition, the actual proximate teratogen may be a metabolite rather than the compound administered. If the moment of final differentiation of a particular organ is known with certainty, then a teratogen must have been present prior to that time, if it is presumed to be the causal agent of the malformation.

During the foetal period the manifestations from toxicological interference are growth retardation, some forms of structural malformations, foetal death, functional impairment and transplacental carcinogenesis. The period of organ and system maturation extends beyond the period of organogenesis and even beyond the prenatal period. Therefore, the susceptible period for the induction of insults that may lead to functional deficits is much longer than that for the induction of gross structural defects. Functions that have been shown to be affected by pre- and early postnatal exposure to chemicals include behaviour, reproduction, endocrine function, immune competence, xenobiotic metabolism, learning capacity and various other physiological functions.

Foetal tissues are intrinsically highly vulnerable to carcinogens because of their high rate of cellular proliferation. This phenomenon has been demonstrated in rats, mice, hamsters, rabbits, pigs, dogs and monkeys. About 30 compounds and groups of chemicals and 12 industrial processes have been shown to induce carcinogenic effects in human beings. However, there is convincing epidemiological evidence of transplacental tumour-induction in humans for only one compound, i.e. diethylstilboestrol (DES). Exposure to DES in utero leads to the development of clear-cell adenocarcinoma of the vagina or cervix in about 1 in

1,000 of those at risk. Moreover, DES is now a recognised female genital tract teratogen. The effects of exposure to DES in utero for males such as infertility are still controversial.

Pharmacokinetics in pregnancy

The metabolisation and kinetics of medicinal products is more complicated in pregnancy than otherwise. In general the effective concentration of a drug or its metabolites is influenced by the following:

- The uptake, distribution, metabolism and excretion by the mother. Changes during pregnancy of some physiologic parameters influencing the metabolisation of chemicals.
- The passage and metabolisation through the yolk sac and the placenta.
- The distribution, metabolism and excretion by the embryo or foetus.
- Re-absorption and swallowing of substances from the amniotic fluid.

However, most of these processes are still unclear and there exists no pharmaceutical product with all these kinetic processes known.

Pregnancy causes physiological changes and adaptations, which can lead to clinically important reductions in the blood concentrations of certain drugs. The total body water increases by as much as 8 liters during pregnancy, which provides a substantially increased volume in which drugs can be distributed. During pregnancy the intestinal, cutaneous and inhalatory absorption of chemicals change due to a decreased peristalsis of the intestines and an increase in skin and lung blood flow. However, this has no consequences for the uptake of medicines from the intestinal tract. Serum proteins relevant to drug binding undergo considerable changes in concentration. Albumin, which binds acidic drugs such as phenytoin, decreases in concentration by up to 10 g/l. The main implication of this change is in the interpretation of drug concentrations. The increased production of female hormones activates enzymes in the maternal liver. This may result in a changed inactivation of medicines. Renal plasma flow would have almost doubled by the last trimester of pregnancy. Drugs that are eliminated unchanged by the kidney are usually eliminated more rapidly, but so far this is shown to be clinically important in only a few cases and make it unnecessary to change the dose of drugs [10] (see Table 1). Some drugs, such as anticonvulsants and theophylline derivatives can undergo changes in distribution and elimination, which lead to ineffective treatment because of inadequate drug concentrations in the blood [11].

Passage of drugs to the unborn and foetal kinetics

Most studies of drug transfer across the maternal and embryonic/foetal barrier are concerned with the end of pregnancy. Little or nothing is known about the transport of substances in the early phases of pregnancy, in which morphologically and functionally both the yolk sac and the placenta develop and change in performance. This is not a major issue with single doses such as with blood products but becomes a matter of concern with long-term therapy. The placenta

Table 1. Changes during pregnancy of the pharmacokinetics of drugs (according to Loebstein [10])

Resorption:	
Gastrointestinal motility	⇩
Lung function	⇧
Skin blood circulation	⇧
Distribution:	
Plasma volume	⇧
Body water	⇧
Plasma protein	⇩
Fat deposition	⇧
Metabolism:	
Liver activity	⇧ ⇩
Excretion:	
Glomerular filtraton	⇧

Table 2. Estimate of causes of developmental disorders (%) (according to Schardein [13], Enders [14], Nelson [15], Wilson [8])

Unknown:	65
Spontaneous developmental disorders	
Multigenetic conditions	
Combinations and interactions of exogenic and endogenic factors	
Genetic diseases	20
Chromosomal disorders	5
Anatomical factors:	2
Uterus anomalies	
Twin pregnancy	
Oligohydramy	
Chemical and physical agents:	4
Medicinal products	
Drugs of abuse (especially alcohol)	
Ionising radiation	
Hyperthermia	
Environmental chemicals	
Maternal conditions:	4
Epilepsy	
Diabetes mellitus	
Hypothyroidism	
Phenylketonuria	
Cytomegaly	
Listeriosis	
Lues	
Rubella	
Toxoplasmosis	
Varicella	

is essentially a lipid barrier between the maternal and embryonic/foetal circulation. Drugs cross the placenta by passive diffusion. A lipid soluble, non-ionised drug of low molecular weight will cross the placenta more rapidly than a more polar drug. Given time, however, most drugs will achieve almost equal concentrations on both sides of the placenta. Thus, the practical view to take in the case of blood donation for a pregnant woman, as recipient is that transfer of biological substances to the foetus is inevitable. However, it has to be understood that an effective concentration might be very low by the technological process in the preparation of the blood products. As will be shown later there exists in this domain of toxicology the phenomenon of a threshold dose under which o detrimental effect is to be expected.

Most drugs have a lower molecular weight than 800 and will therefore be able to cross the placenta. The notable exceptions to this rule are conjugated steroid and peptide hormones such as insulin and growth hormone. In the third month of pregnancy the foetal liver is already capable of activating or inactivating chemical substances through oxidation [12]. In the foetal compartment detoxification of drugs and their metabolites takes place at a low level, certainly in the first half of pregnancy. This aspect among others, such as excretion in the amniotic fluid, makes it understandable that accumulation of biological active substances might take place in the foetal compartment. The not yet existing blood/brain barrier in the foetus is another characteristic that might be of importance for possible foetotoxic effects of chemicals.

Causes of developmental disorders

Wilson, during a presentation in Vienna in 1973 [8], presented an estimate of the causes of developmental disorders (Table 2). His most important observation, that about two third of the causes are of unknown aetiology, is still valuable. This lack of clear causal connections explains the problems faced in primary prevention of developmental disorders.

Medicinal products and other chemical substances are estimated to account for only 4%, but they may play a more important role in the causation of developmental defects through interaction with other factors and maternal metabolic diseases. Antenatal care, including prenatal screening and diagnosis are valuable tools in this respect. Table 3 presents an overview of the drugs and chemicals proven to be developmental toxicants in humans.

Embryo/foetotoxic risk assessment

There are different methods for assessing the embryo/foetotoxicity of medicinal products. The risk assessment process for new drugs is limited to experimental studies on laboratory animals. For drugs on the market, large epidemiological studies are of great value. In the case of thalidomide more than two years passed before Dr Lenz' early suspicions about the phocomelia-tragedy [7] had to be accepted by his opponents.

It is generally accepted that the predictive value of animal teratogenicity and reproductive toxicity tests in extrapolating results of chemicals into terms of human safety is less than adequate. Hence, it can be understood that not all

Table 3. Medicinal products, chemicals and drugs of abuse with proven embryo-/foeto-toxic potential in humans*

Agent	Indicating signs
ACE-inhibitors	Anuria
Alcohol	Foetal alcohol syndrome/effects
Androgens	Masculinisation
Antimetabolites	Multiple malformations
Benzodiazepines	Floppy infant syndrome
Lead	Cognitive developmental retardation
Carbamazepine†	Spina bifida, multiple malformations
Coumarin anticoagulants	Coumarine syndrome
Diethylstilboestrol	Vaginal dysplasia and neoplasms
Ionising radiation	Microcephaly, leukaemia
Iodine overdose	Reversible hypothyroidism
Cocain	CNS-, intestinal- and kidney damage
Methylmercury	Cerebral palsy, mental retardation
Misoprostol	Moebius-sequence, reduction of extremities
Polychlorbiphenyls	Mental retardation, immunological disorders, skin discoloration
Penicillamin	Cutis laxa
Phenobarbital/Primidon† (anticonvulsive dose)	Multiple malformations
Phenytoin†	Multiple malformations
Retinoids	Ear, CNS, cardiovascular and skeletal disorders
Tetracycline (after week 15)	Discoloration of teeth
Thalidomide	Malformations of extremities a.o.
Trimethadione	Multiple malformations
Valproic acid†	Spina bifida, multiple malformations
Vitamin A‡ (>25.000 IU/day)	See retinoids

* Individual risk is dose- and time-dependent. Risk increase with monotherapy or single administration of most substances in list only two- to threefold at maximum (see text). Never use this list for individual risk characterisation or risk management!

† Combination therapy may increase the teratogenic risk substantially.

‡ Prevent exposure to >10,000 IU/day. Provitamine A = Beta-Carotene is known to be harmless

developmental toxic substances were discovered by laboratory screening methods before they were used in humans.

With the exception of androgens, several anti-mitotic drugs, sodium valproate and vitamin A-derivatives, all human teratogens were discovered earlier in man than in animals. Most of these discoveries were made from case studies by alert clinicians and not primarily from epidemiological studies. Specific epidemiological examination in prospective cohort, or retrospective case-control studies (see below) might provide the final evidence of such hypotheses (postmarketing surveillance).

In this respect it is worth mentioning that in the 1970s collaboration was started among birth defects registries around the world. At present, this International Clearinghouse for Birth Defects Monitoring Systems consists of birth defects surveillance programs, monitoring several millions new-borns each year. Co-operative research is performed, but the main activity is the exchange of information collected within each program. An important aim is a world wide surveillance. A primary goal of the Clearinghouse is to detect changes in the incidence of specific malformations or patterns of malformations that may indicate the presence of chemicals, including medicinal hazards, to identify such hazards, and – if possible – to eliminate them.

The process of assessing a reproductive or embryo/foetoxic effect of a drug includes the establishment of a biological plausibility and epidemiological evidence (see criteria according to Shepard [16] 1994 and Wilson [8]1977 in Table 4).

Table 4. The process of assessing a reproductive or embryo/foetoxic effect of a drug includes the establishment of a biological plausibility and epidemiological evidence with the following criteria (according to Shepard [16] and Wilson [8])

A sudden increase in the prevalence of a specific malformation is observed.
An association is established between the introduction or an increased usage of a drug and an increased prevalence of a specific malformation in a certain region and during a given time.
Drug use must have taken place in the sensitive period for the induction of that specific malformation.
The drug or its metabolite suspected of causing the malformation has to be proved capable of reaching the embryo or foetus.
It must be established that the drug and not the condition for which the drug is prescribed causes the specific malformation.
The findings have to be confirmed by another independent study.
The results of specific laboratory animal studies might support the epidemiological findings.

The prolonged use of medicines during pregnancy occurs in cases of chronic (metabolic) diseases such as epilepsy, psychiatric illnesses, diabetes, thyroid dysfunction etc. There are clear indications of developmental toxicity amongst these groups of medicines and epidemiological investigations deserve a high priority. Greater uniformity in prescribing habits would enhance the likelihood of detecting causal factors of developmental disorders. The registration of new drugs developed for conditions requiring treatment during pregnancy should be based on comparative clinical trials in which not only the therapeutic but also the teratogenic properties are examined.

In 1990 two networks of Teratology Information Services were established: one in the Americas OTIS (Organization of Teratology Information Services) and another in Europe ENTIS (European Network of Teratology Information Services). A teratology information service provides health professionals and patients with a 'tailor-made' information relating to the pertinent situation, illness and chemical exposure of the person involved. These services also carry out follow-up studies (case-registry studies, prospective cohort-control studies) to learn about what happened during the course of pregnancy and the health of the new born.

As earlier mentioned developmental disorders are not only manifested as structural malformations – other embryo/foetotoxic effects are:

- Spontaneous abortions;
- Intrauterine growth retardation;
- Reversible functional postnatal effects, such as sedation, hypoglycaemia, bradycardia and withdrawal effects;
- Central nervous system disorders, from motility disturbances to learning disabilities;
- Immunological disturbances; and
- Fertility and reproductive problems.

Most of these are not apparent at birth but will be manifested much later. This explains why the prevalence of developmental disorders is about 3% at birth and at about 8% the age of 5 years.

Classification of drugs used in pregnancy

About 80 % of pregnant women use prescribed or over-the-counter drugs. There is no doubt that, even in pregnancy, drugs are often unjustifiably used. Health care professionals and pregnant women need to develop a more critical attitude to the use of drugs during pregnancy, or more importantly to the use of drugs during the fertile period. These drugs should only be taken when essential, thereby avoiding many unnecessary and unknown risks. The same obviously applies for social drugs like tobacco, alcohol and addictive drugs.

Since 1984, classification systems have been introduced in the USA, Sweden and Australia. Classification is general and has a 'ready-made' fashion. These systems allow a general estimation of the safety of drugs in pregnancy and to reproduction. The FDA classification is at this moment in 'reconstruction'. In the European Community (EC) a specification (in specified wording) of the medicinal products to be used in pregnancy has to be given on the summary of product characteristics including:

- Facts on human experience and conclusions from pre-clinical toxicity studies which are of relevance for the assessment of risks associated with exposure during pregnancy;
- Recommendations on the use of the medicinal product at different times during pregnancy in respect of gestation; and
- Recommendations on the management of the situation of an inadvertent exposure, where relevant.

Alternative remedies

There has been scarcely any systematic study of alternative remedies such as homeopathics with respect to their tolerability during pregnancy. However there are no case reports on embryo- or foetotoxic effects after maternal intake of recommended doses.

In the case of phytotherapeutics, therapeutic doses should be adhered to and teas should not be used excessively. Plant preparations (in high doses) are not always harmless. If there is a choice, non-alcoholic preparations are preferable. More or less commonly used, in particular, are valerian, hops and kawain (kavapyrone from the kava-kava root) for nervousness and sleep disturbances, echinacea as an immune stimulant, ginko biloba to improve general circulation, ginseng to improve performance, aescin-preparations (horse chestnut extract) for vein problems, agnus castus (monk's pepper) for gynaecological indications, hypericin (St. John's Wort) for depressive mood, and mistletoe as supportive anti-cancer therapy. Systematic studies on these phytotherapeutics in pregnancy are lacking, but no damage to the foetus has, as yet, been described when administration remained in a normal range.

Paternal use of medicinal products

Husbands or partners are rarely, if ever, admonished to avoid known embryo/foetotoxic medicinal products. Nevertheless, evidence is slowly accumulating that if males are exposed to reproductive agents the prevalence of birth defects among their offspring may be increased. So far no one is certain about the safety of substances that after administration or via occupational exposure to males can cause birth defects. Theoretically three possible causes can be given:

- substances, such as cytostatics could damage the sperm itself genetically, impair spermatogenesis or the maturation of sperm;
- agents might act through the semen. Many substances are excreted in semen and are present along with the sperm before, during but also (long) after the moment of conception; and
- effects of the toxic agents could be produced indirectly as a result of the action of, for example, drugs in the male.

No one believes at this moment that medicinal products taken by males and also not substances through blood products from these persons are a major contribution to developmental disorders, but many investigators conclude that these medicinal products through this route could cause disorders. Such possible cause of developmental toxicity is essential and should not be forgotten, when stimulating primary prevention of congenital disorders.

References

1. Schaefer Chr. ed. Drugs during pregnancy and lactation, Amsterdam, Elsevier, 2001.
2. Chamberlain G. Organisation of antenatal care. BMJ 1991;302:647.
3. Warkany J, Nelson RC. Appearance of skeletal abnormalities in the offspring of rats retarded on a deficient diet. Science 1940;92:383-84.
4. Barker DJP. Mothers, babies and health in later life. Churchill Livingston, Edinburgh 1998, 2nd edition.
5. Hale F. Pigs born without eyeballs. J Hered 1933;24:105-06.

6. Gregg NM. Congenital cataract following German measles in mother. Trans Ophthalmol Soc Aust 1941;3:35-46.
7. Lenz W. Kindliche Fehlbildungen nach Medikament während der Gravidität? Dtsch Med Wochenschr 1961;86:2555-56.
8. Wilson JD. Embryotoxicity of drugs to man. In: Handbook of teratology, Vol. 1. Wilson JD, Frazer FC, eds.. New York, Plenum Press, 1977;309-55.
9. Committee on Dev. Toxicol. NAS/NRC. Scientific Frontiers in Developmental Toxicology and Risk Assessment. National Research Council, Washington DC 2000;10-25.
10. Loebstein R, Lalkin A, Koren G. Pharmacokinetic changes during pregnancy and their clinical relevance. Clin Pharmacokinet 1997;33:328-43.
11. Lander CM, Smith MT, Chalk JB et al. Bioavailability in pharmacokinetics of phenytoin during pregnancy. Eur J Clin Pharmacol 1984;27:105-10.
12. Juchau MR. Bioactivation in chemical teratogenesis. Ann Rev Pharmacol Toxicol 1989; 29:165-87.
13. Schardein JL. Chemically induced birth defects. New York, Marcel Dekker, 2000, 4th edition.
14. Enders G. Infektionen und Impfungen in der Schwangerschaft. München, Urban & Schwarzenberg, 1991, 2nd edition.
15. Nelson K, Holmes LB. Malformations due to presumed spontaneous mutations in newborn infants. N Engl J Med 1989;320:19-23.
16. Shepard TH. Letter: "proof" of teratogenicity. Teratology 1994;50:97.

Electronic database offering an overview on published studies.
Reprotox. Information database on environmental hazards to human reproduction and development. Quarterly updated. Reproductive Toxicology Center (RTC).
Columbia Hospital for Women Medical Center, 2440 M Street, NW, Ste 217. Washington, D.C. 20037-1404, Telephone +001-202-293-5137.

DISCUSSION

Moderators: R.Y. Dodd and C.Th. Smit Sibinga

R.Y. Dodd (Rockville, MD, USA): Dr. van der Poel, I often wonder really how we demonstrate the value of donor questions. A couple of things stand out in my mind. One is that if you take a look at individuals who declare themselves to be unsuitable as donors - and there are a number of ways of doing this - there is actually a very low risk associated with this group of people. Furthermore, the actual number of donors who are rejected as a result of questioning is extraordinarily low and there seems to be something of a paradox here. My own feeling is that the fact that questions are to be asked has some impact on whether or not people turn up to donate. But would you like to elaborate a little bit on what I think is a paradox.

C.L. van der Poel (Amsterdam, NL): I as well think it is paradoxical. What I noticed in the past, was that rejection as a donor is very awkward, no matter what the reason is. One takes time to come and one has to wait. When this ends up in deferral, this is really awkward. Second, it is not only awkward when it regards a question which relates to a risk for the recipient like an infection of HIV or hepatitis. It also includes a risk for oneself as well. So, not only do you have to be very honest, you also have to accept that you may be a risk for others. It requires intelligence to understand that there is a wide area of non-specificity about these questions and to be able to rationalize. So, I think it regards a certain subset of donors who would be willing to say 'yes I carry that risk, so I stop. I cannot donate'. We have not really studied that; there is no study as far as I know about the profile of donors who positively answer these questions. First, there are the donors who deny the questions. Second there are the donors whom you counsel when you find them infected. Indeed it is very threatening to have a risk factor and when you then are counseled for your. We have seen that in the US and that has been published extensively[1]. So, there might be studies needed on the mechanisms why those two different sets of population actually occur.

R.Y. Dodd: I have nothing to add. I think that is a very interesting analysis. I do think those studies need to be done. The problem is that you really have to sample the rejected donors routinely and that is not an easy thing to do.

---

1. Van der Poel CL, Cuypers, HTM, Reesink HW et al. Risk factors in HCV infected blood donors. Transfusion 1991;31:777-79.

M. Postma (Groningen, NL): Dr. van der Poel, I was very impressed with the residual risk estimates for the different viruses you showed for the Netherlands. I knew that these kinds of estimates were available for Germany, USA, but I wondered about the level of evidence for the Netherlands of these estimates. Are these estimates your highly valued expert opinion or are studies under way to be published?

C.L. van der Poel: Well, this is really a challenge; should I publish? Actually, they are published in our annual report, where we give the incidence. So there are two parameters you always look at: First is the prevalence in new donors, a cross section of the population; what do you find when you first test a population. This can only be done in new donors. The first time tested persons provide the prevalence, the cross section of the population you sample. That is not the real risk, the real risk is in the incidence. How many donors get sick, get infected during their career as a donor. That is were the risk assessment comes from. Actually this has been calculated by the model used by George Schreiber[1]. To be honest there are a many things you could say about that model. It is very simple; it says the residual risk is the incidence times the donation interval as a fraction of the year. It turns out that people who are infected with HIV for instance have a longer interval before they donate this positive donation. For hepatitis C probably not, for those are people who usually remain non-symptomatic. For hepatitis B it might be as well, because some of these people do not feel well. So, we have to study that in a model and I know you are an expert in models and I am not. So, I leave the epidemiology at this edge.

J.H. Marcelis (Eindhoven, NL): Prof. Peters, you started your lecture by raising the question whether donations from donors who are on medication or have drug abuse transfused to pregnant women have a negative result on the offspring of the recipients. At the final part of your lecture you talked about accutane and as far as I know accutane is a psoralen is that true? In the Netherlands, as you may know, there is currently research ongoing in blood technology to add psoralens to blood products to kill all viruses and all bacteria. It is not only the donor who is a risk factor for our blood product when using drugs, but we ourselves are probably the biggest risk by adding this kind of drug to our products. Could you comment on that, please?

R.Y. Dodd: Dr. Wages is going to respond to that comment and rightly so. I think that this kind of question does generate a certain amount of concern in the face of what we just heard from Mr. de Wit about the European attitude towards pathogen inactivation. In fact, the actual risk of an adverse outcome from transfusion transmissible agents is negligible. The question really is how can you establish that the potential adverse effects of a treated product are less than those of what it is trying to prevent. Certainly, you are never going to be able to show

1. Schreiber GB, Bush MP, Kleinman SH, Korelitz JJ. The risk of transfusion- transmitted viral infections. The Retrovirus Epidemiology Donor Study. N Engl J Med 1996; 334:1685-90.

that in clinical trials on five or six hundred patients, where you would at worst find a 1% adverse effect outcome. Dr. Wages really should have the final word on this particular question.

D. S. Wages (Concord, CA, USA): Just a comment on the previous question and also a further question for Dr. Peters. I work for a company, Cerus Corporation, that is developing a new system for pathogen inactivation which does introduce a psoralen that specifically synthesized a non-natural psoralen for pathogen inactivation. In the process of developing this compound, the standard toxicological assays for safety and tolerability have been done in a variety of animal models that are common to all drugs introduced into humans. Although I am not an organic chemist I believe the actual structure of the psoralen S59 is substantially different from accutane. My question for Dr. Peters is that given what you described to us for the evaluability of compounds and their ability to cause teratogenic changes during pregnancy, what confidence can we have for any type of new introduced compounds? That would not have to be drugs, it can be any type of new food, a new food additive, anything in the environment that one would not be currently taking, could pose a risk for introducing teratological changes. I guess, perhaps, as a follow up in addition to that question would be: How common are truly teratological toxic agents in the environment?

P.W.J. Peters (Utrecht, NL): Thank you for that question, because one of the issues, which I did not mention, is the detection methods of new teratogens. Of course, post marketing surveillance is the first answer but that is difficult. I mentioned the birth defect detecting systems, but they mostly do not register a drug intake and probably never blood donation. So that is really a problem. There is, however, another system both in the Americas and Europe; these systems are called OTIS and ENTIS. In Europe: the European Network Teratology Information Service. They build case registries of pregnancies with drug treatment and they perform follow up studies to ascertain the health of the newborn. Then the data from different teratology information services are collected in order to learn about the possibility that a substance introduced on the market might cause a defect.

We understood from the thalidomide disaster that it took many years before the substance could be identified as causing such problems. Thus post marketing surveillance is the easy answer; the difficulty is to do it.

J.H. Marcelis: As I understand, women who get accutane must be prepared not to become pregnant for at least two years. Is that the time you need to eliminate all your vitamin A.

P.W.J. Peters: Here is a confusion. Hypervitaminosis A and also hypovitaminosis A might cause birth defects. Roaccutane is a Vitamin A-derivative that has a completely different developmental toxic pattern. The problem is that it does not metabolize and is not detoxified that quickly as Vitamin A. That is the reason that you need to abstain from pregnancy after the last use of the substance such a long time. This is an example of what I meant: it all depends on the characteristics of the substance and the concentrations.

J.P.H.B. Sybesma (Dordrecht, NL): Dr. van der Poel, I was surprised you showed that there were more possibilities to have plasmapheresis when you had no paid donors. Because of course some people and some countries say that you need paid donors otherwise you do no get enough plasma. I can understand that when you have in one country both systems that the people that do not get paid say well do it yourself, because I do not want to co-operate. So, I want to know in what country you had more possibilities when you did not pay the donor.

C.L. van der Poel: I have been looking for that in the PubMed Database, but it is really difficult to find data on this. We know that there have been third world countries where they shifted from paid plasma donor system to a voluntary non-paid system. Actually after that the blood supply went better. What I was referring to is actually a paper by Paul Holland in Transfusion 1994[1], where he quotes Harvey Klein, who has personal data from the NIH blood center. In 1984 the payment for cytapheresis – which was logical then in 1984 as cytapheresis takes a long time – so there was some payment, because he felt mandated to stop. So, there was a group of donors who would donate and got some payment and he stopped paying. The message is, it did not negatively effect his donor base.

C.Th. Smit Sibinga (Groningen, NL): Dr. Dodd, when you described the histories of hepatitis B, hepatitis C and HIV in your marvelous presentation, what – if you would use just a few sentences – would be *the* lessons learned?

R.Y. Dodd: I think that the biggest lesson in the long term was that all of these measures that were undertaken were actually based on good epidemiologic science not necessarily directed towards blood safety. I think that is a very important message for all of us to look broadly at the issues involved. Not necessarily to try to seek our own solutions but rather to be expert in implementing the solutions that have been partially developed by others. I am sure there are many other lessons, but I think that that is an important one. Keep science in there, keep it vital, keep your eyes open and work hard at implementing the lessons.

C.Th. Smit Sibinga: That is a very important answer. Could I then extend that question to Dr. van der Poel and ask: What is the actual science behind a number of the questions we ask our donors for selection.

C.L. van der Poel: That depends on the question, which is asked. This is not political but reality.

---

1. Holland PV. Paid cytapheresis sellers, not donors. Letter to the editor. Transfusion 1994;34:836

C.Th. Smit Sibinga: Let us focus on the teratogenic effects. The use of medication that might cause a deleterious effect under defined conditions in a specific patient.

C.L. van der Poel: My recollection is about ro-accutane and all those newer compounds like tigason and neo-tigason. Actually, there was a debate when the agent was used widely with youngsters for acne. You get a number of people who actually use it. Then there were questions whether or not this was teratogenic for the recipient when the donor would donate and be under this drug, given the fact that the half time is very long. So, those drugs were actually the only ones put on that list because then it was questioned to the manufacturer 'can you be sure?' The manufacturer would say 'you cannot give it to pregnant women'. So, that is where it started. Now I have had several sessions, and I am not exaggerating it has been years and years and over an over again. Young and critical and educated doctors come up with the whole book of drugs of the Netherlands. We get some more of these drugs which might have the same effect, and then what are you saying to that – I have no answer. This is how it went and actually the problem is, there is no evidence behind it. There was just a reasoning behind it and the reasoning could be done for the whole list. Maybe, we should use the expertise of Prof. Peters to go through the whole list. He might say 'well, maybe yes, maybe not' and he would end up with a long list where he would say 'I do not know'.

R.Y. Dodd: I think that Dr. Smit Sibinga has raised a very interesting question. Dr. van der Poel has given an interesting answer as well. But the fact of the matter is that many of the questions that we ask, we ask in the absence of science, as a substitute for technology that we would like to use. We could probably agree if we had testing that was a hundred percent effective, we might be less interested in questioning. Even in the world of perfect testing or perfect inactivation, I think that the FDA would still like us to prevent potentially infectious donors from coming into the system for two reasons. One is that there is a risk of laboratory error and the other is that there is a potential exposure of the staff in the blood center. So, there is kind of a rationale to continue but it is not a very good one. I think it is reasonable to ask how many questions do we still need, how many questions could be eliminated without any significant impact. We could probably think of quite a few, but unfortunately in many places these got written into law and law is hard to change – much harder than science.

C.Th. Smit Sibinga: That is very true

P.W.J. Peters: Perhaps an addition, just a suggestion: while you are not far away from clinical pharmacology, why would it not be possible, that blood levels are checked in patients who use certain drugs and certainly in patients with a chronic medication to learn how much of the substance is present.

P.J.M. van den Burg (Amsterdam, NL): Dr. Peters, do you suggest that all donors who use medication should be deferred as blood donor? Because, if you look at enclosures for medicine a number of drugs have the message that it could generate a teratogenic effect. We only have deferral for a small number of drugs like ro-accutane and tigason. How can we cope with the problem?

P.W.J. Peters: There are two types of lists or perhaps three. One is the list of substances, which we have made indicating that there is no risk at all. The drugs that we use preferably in pregnancy. The other list consists of drugs with proven pharmacological effects; the third suggests that these drugs might cause developmental defects.

D.S. Wages: Prof. Peters, has there ever been a documented case where a pregnant patient received a blood transfusion and then had a birth defect in the child subsequent to the transfusion that could definitively be ascribed to the blood transfusion.

P.W.J. Peters: The answer is: not to my knowledge. But I say to my knowledge and I must say I have never studied this per se. Of course, in preparing this lecture I have talked to a lot reproductive and developmental toxicologists and pharmacologists. They were not aware of such a case and they might be the persons who might have the most experience. Also I have sent around a message to the colleagues at the teratology information service in Europe: 'Are you aware of such a case?' The answer was: 'No'. But even that does not say much, because this is just not really studied. I asked for case reports; there are no well-performed studies. But be aware of something else. Why do transfusions take place during pregnancy. This means that there must be an underlying illness, perhaps a surgery. We know that many situations a problem in pregnancy itself could induce all types of defects. So, that is another problem. I do not think that in a case where there is a malformation one would think immediately and make the association with blood transfusion.

H.J.C. de Wit (Amsterdam, NL): Additional to part of the discussion that it might be useful to ask the question now. Dr. Dodd, as you said we prefer scientific basis for donor questionnaires. If you do not have a test for a potential transmissible disease the first thing you should do is exclude donors on epidemiological grounds. So, the question of excluding donors on the basis of their consumption habits might be a hot issue because prion disease is theoretically transmissible by blood transfusion. Now the question would be: In the United States the FDA implemented a ban on British donors, so exclusion of donors that lived in the United Kingdom including the Channel Islands between 1980 and 1996 for more then six months. At that time the FDA could state that the risk reduction achieved with that question was about 95% or 97%. The question is whether this ban on British donors is going to be extended to Western Europe. There is a draft guideline from FDA and this will be in debate again in January 2002. That would mean that in fact all Europeans would be banned from giving blood in the United States. What is the scientific basis behind this discussion and could you tell anything about the added safety – more than 97% – to the theoretical risk?

R.Y. Dodd: Dr. van der Poel is whispering "precautionary principle" in my ear. I think that this has been an extremely difficult situation for regulators. I believe that actually one of the first things that motivated regulators outside the United Kingdom were the actions that the United Kingdom itself took in some of these fields. For example the United Kingdom elected no longer to fractionate own plasma. I think that if you talk carefully to the British and the British regulators about this it was more of a pragmatic move than a safety move, because of the difficulties of recalling plasma containing materials from all over the world. Nevertheless, this was seen by regulators as a safety oriented movement. They clearly heard that the British regard their own plasma as inappropriate for inclusion in pool products. So, what does a regulator in the United States or in Australia or many other countries do with this piece of information? I think all the rest, when you talk about science, really boils down not so much to the science as to the underlying assumptions that are made around these regulatory postures. When you say that the FDA made some estimates of benefits, yes indeed they did. These estimates were based on questionnaire based studies on donors that determined how long different donors had spent in different areas that might have been effected by BSE or potentially by vCJD. The concept there was a very simple one, it was really the only one that could be used and that is the longer you were in a place where you might have been exposed the higher the likelihood that you yourself are infectious, The FDA actually applied again some fairly arbitrary – but I want to say sophisticated – but thoughtful modeling to the data that they had in hand. Their thinking and doing of all this was on the basis of beef exports, cattle feed exports and appearance of the bovine disease. If you take the risk as one hundred in the UK, in France perhaps now it is five (and this is actually born out by cases of vCJD) and in the rest of Europe about 1.5. They also had some additions for American servicemen stationed in Europe who had been fed with British beef. This is where you can challenge the model. In fact my own organization has challenged the model and basically says any exposure needs to be dealt with. In fact that policy is probably as good as any other. So, it is very hard to tease out the science here and the precautionary principle is riding.

J. Verburg (Hoogeveen, NL): About cost effectiveness, I have another question also in that area. I am very interested in hearing all those things about medicines they give influence on embryonic development and so on. I think in the way we are speaking about it, it is so theoretically and so very difficult to discover as Prof. Peters tells us. He showed us many problems and showed us how difficult it is to find out whether there is any influence of those medicines on the born children. I wonder whether it would not be better to give instructions to the doctors to be very careful on giving transfusions to people, especially to women in their fertile age. I tried to give some instructions to young doctors in our hospitals. Anytime I do that and I tell them about the risks of transfusions they are so confused, they do not know anything about it, really. So, I think we should start with that; just tell them what are the risks. We are talking about the unknown risks.

C.L. van der Poel: Most complications of blood transfusion are not related to hepatitis C or HIV infections, not even to theoretical risks of other agents. They are associated with giving the wrong blood or they are associated to a lesser extent to bacterial contamination. I am very glad that we could convince with scientific data the minister that we can implement bacterial testing of platelets because that is really a risk. Now in terms of your question not to use too much blood, the use of red cells in the Netherlands has gone down considerably over the last two years. Actually, consumption went down with a hundred thousand units per year, because there is an increasing awareness among clinicians that you could transfuse much less than before. This is also addressed by a recent consensus meeting which is set up by the CBO. They will come out with a consensus about transfusion practice taking into account all of these issues like optimal use, what is the risk and how do we set up a hemovigilance system to really know what the risks are. But you already know from data from other countries that the risks are not in the risks that I presented, which are very popular. I think you are right, you could do much on the risks and mistakes in a clinical setting. But it is a very difficult area. For instance it was very difficult to convince the European Union that in the coming Directive there should be a paragraph saying that the side effects of transfusions should be reported. Because it was felt that that part of the transfusion chain was not relevant. It is all about blood establishments like Sanquin or other systems, while the real safety lies in the clinic. I think you are very right and Sanquin and myself and anybody you could ask in the blood system in the Netherlands would be very happy to help in educating young doctors and preferably with the new consensus coming out.

C.Th. Smit Sibinga: It is even better to educate the older doctors.

To complement this information which Dr. van der Poel just has given, as you have seen from my presentation on behalf of Dr. Gaby Vercauteren, WHO is giving a lot of attention at this point of time to the rational use of human blood. Last year in the July issue of Transfusion Today, as a supplement a set of recommendations was published of an important WHO meeting which was undertaken by the Europe Region Office in Copenhagen[1]. The meeting took place in London on this issue splitting it into what would be regarded the rationale in the surgical field, in anesthesiology, in pediatrics, in hematology and so forth. There is a follow-up meeting which will be held end of October here in Groningen to further elaborate on these recommendations, which relate to educate prescribing clinicians and designing clinical indicators.[2]

T. Smith (Girvan, Scotland): It struck me that we unfortunately and tragically have an ongoing study of deaths from CJD in the United Kingdom. We have 101 deaths and six more I believe who are in the process of dying from the disease. Has anyone studied the number of these people who have had blood trans-

1. Transfusion Today 2000;43 (supplement).
2. Development of Quality Systems to Improve the Clinical Use of Blood. Report of a WHO Regional Workshop, Groningen 2001. WHO EURO, Copenhagen 2002. (EUR/01/5016767).

fusions? That is, the proportion of them who have had blood transfusions in comparison to the proportion of the people in the general public who have had blood transfusions and whether these proportions are different? Is it too early yet, or are the numbers too small? Would this give an idea whether blood transfusion has any influence on CJD?

C.L. van der Poel: Maybe I could answer part of the question. There has been a case control study on classical CJD on a European scale. However, there was no significance between the arms; so, there was no difference in receiving transfusion versus non receiving. The power of that study was questioned, given the low prevalence one might need a very big study. The other thing is that about 104 patients in the United Kingdom to my knowledge are followed up in a registry. The scientific committee on spongiform encephalopathy in Edinburgh has a registry of all those persons and as soon as there is a match between a variant CJD case and recipient of a product that will be noticed. So, there is a system in place to follow that up. My present concern is about – but this is not proven – neurosurgical interventions rather than transfusion.

T. Smith: I was wondering about recipients; how many of these present-day patients or people who have died from CJD have received blood transfusions before they got CJD? Is there any evidence on that and whether that differs from the general population?

R.Y. Dodd: Well, I think Dr. van der Poel is absolutely correct that there have been two case control studies relating to classical CJD. There have also been some look back studies, one in Europe and one in the United States, in which individuals who have given blood and were subsequently found to have developed CJD became the starting point for look back investigations in which all their prior donations were tracked back to patients. The patients have been looked at in one of a number of ways. For example in the United States an ongoing study looked at 23 such donors and 300 of their recipients. Something over 1000 person years of follow-up has been accumulated on patients who died: no death were due to neurological disease. The others as far as is known are healthy and not yet sick. Now that is a very small number but it is better than nothing. With respect to vCJD in the UK there is a very elaborate programme which looks at cases and evaluates the donors to those cases; it looks at cases and determines whether they have been donors and if so tracks the recipients of those donors. That involves a lot of between different agencies and some pretty heavy ethical considerations are involved. But I think that it is pretty clear this ongoing study will be of value.

C.L. van der Poel: About the frequency – the point of your question was also whether there were more recipients of blood among the vCJD patients. I recall a talk of Herbert Budka in Vienna[1]. I thought it was at that time a hundred and

1. Budka H. Prions and transfusion medicine. State-of-the-Art paper. Vox Sang 2000; 78(Suppl 2):231-38.

three patients in total, including the probable cases and I think they had 7 recipients of blood, which frequency in my opinion would not sound different from a general population.

C.Th. Smit Sibinga: We had a very interesting start of this 26th symposium. To close I would go back to Prof. Peters defining the human species in differing from other species. Looking each other in the face – he said – is one of the major discriminative functions. Another function is what we actually traced in between the lines here: Using our intellectual capacity in raising questions. The only species that really can raise questions, raises them loudly. That is where actually the positive side of our species is, because once we raise questions we have to come up with answers. Usually we do not come up with proper answers, let it be science based answers. We come up with anecdotal answers and that is what basically leads us into today's problems in blood transfusion.

II. TRANSMISSIBLE DISEASES

BACTERIAL CONTAMINATION OF BLOOD AND BLOOD PRODUCTS
AN UNDERESTIMATED PROBLEM

Jan H. Marcelis[1]

Introduction

From the very beginning of transfusion practice bacterial sepsis due to blood transfusion was recognized. Currently the frequency of bacterial sepsis attributable to transfusion of contaminated blood products appears to be similar to that of transfusion-associated hepatitis C infections, but higher than for infections with Hepatitis B or HIV.

Whole blood is a well-known nutrient and is able together with additives like citrate and glucose to support bacterial multiplication. Thus active research should be carried out to focus on innovative measures to detect and eliminate infected units before transfusion.

Prevalence

Overall about 0.4% of all blood products are contaminated with bacteria. Morrow [1] and Blajchman [2] estimated that about 5% of these products will result in manifest transfusion transmitted bacterial infections (TTI). From 1994 to 1996 The French Hemovigilance system reported 43 TTI, of whom 14 patients died. The relative risk for TTI is the highest in platelet concentrates [3]. In 16% of the patients in the USA who died after transfusion a relation with bacterial contamination was established [4]. In the UK, the SHOT (Serious Hazard Of Transfusion) project reported from 1985 till 1998 28 fatal casualties; (in the same period 2 HIV sero-negative donors with a window-donation were reported [5]. In the Netherlands we found that 0,36% of about 1900 whole blood units were contaminated with bacteria [6]. Platelets were contaminated in 1.8% (n= 2430) [7]. Most authors report that platelet concentrates are more contaminated than red cells [8].

Transfusion transmitted infections caused by bacteria

Clinical signs suggesting a TTI are listed in Table 1. The frequency of nonfatal outcome of TTI is not well characterized because heavily transfused patients mostly have illnesses with high mortality rates of their own. The majority of clinical symptoms are attributed to the patient's immune response to transfused leukocytes, or to the underlying disease often with similar presentation. The risk

1. Medical microbiologist, Sanquin Division Blood Bank De Meierij, Eindhoven, NL.

Table 1. Clinical signs in transfusion transmitted diseases

Fever (>38.5°C)
Rigors
Tachycardia
Hypotension
Nausea, vomiting
Abdominal pain
Low back pain
Shock
Oliguria
Transfusion related
Mortality rate up to 26%

to overlook TTI grows the more time has elapsed between blood transfusion and clinical signs resulting in an underestimation the problem.

A TTI is established when the same bacteria are isolated from the blood product (and preferably related products from the same donation) and from blood cultures taken from the patient. Positive blood cultures from a patient can also originate from another infective focus. Especially when coagulase negative staphylococci are isolated extensive testing has to be done to exclude that they originate from the patient's skin instead of the blood product [9]. When the patient become unwell during a transfusion often the procedure is stopped abruptly and aseptically disconnection of the blood bag is not carried out properly. As a result the blood product can be contaminated by the patients' own blood leading to false positive results [10].

Gram-negative bacteria more often result in sepsis due to the transfused cell wall lipopolysaccharide, whereas Gram-positive bacteria result in more mild infections. About 10^4 coagulase negative staphylococci (CNS) are easily tolerated and cleared by most patients [11]. Patients undergoing marrow ablative therapy are in bad condition and are transfused with large number of platelet units. These patients are therefore in great risk for TTI even at low bacterial numbers [12,13]. Intravascular prosthetic devices and grafts are at risk for colonization by "non pathogenic" Gram-positive skin flora, which could lead to the necessity of removing them [14]. For high-risk recipients cellular blood components completely free from bacteria are advised [15].

Microorganisms and source

In most cases bacterial contamination of blood products originates from the donor. Most important is the phlebotomy site. The superficial human skin is colonized with bacteria up to 10^6/mm2. Also the deeper skin-levels are colonized with bacteria. Proper disinfection can reduce the number to 10^3, but no matter how carefully blood is drawn, there is no way to completely avoid introduction of microbes. While penetrating the skin many needles are liable to excise fragments entering the blood bag at the beginning of the donation [16,17].

Discarding the first 10–15 ml of a donation (with skin fragments) can reduce the number of bacteria [18-20]. A second source is bacteremia occurring for instance after dental procedures [21] and in cases of chronic sub clinical infections (low-grade osteomyelitis, gastroenteritis, Lyme disease, *Erlichia* etc) [22]. In most cases however donor anamnesis will reveal cryptic infection thus preventing donation.

At temperatures above 17°C leukocytes are able to phagocytose and kill bacteria even after the donation, but this holds not for all microorganisms [23,24]. Filtration of whole blood after about 6–8 hours is able to remove free and phagocytosed bacteria [25]. In red cells storage (at 4°C) will result in further reduction because this is far beyond optimal temperature of the human commensal flora (mesophilics). Also improper preparation procedures, manufacturing deficiencies or storage conditions of blood products, bags and filtration units environmental contaminants may result in contamination [26]. Finally blood products can be contaminated during sampling for bacterial culture.

In red cells Gram-negative aerobe microorganisms seem of most clinical importance [13]. When stored for longer periods bacteria able to multiply at 4°C (psychrophilics), like yersinea and pseudomonas are associated with infections. In the Netherlands we detected a Gram-negative bacterium only once in about 25,000 whole blood samples [19].Yersinea infections are rarely seen in Dutch hospitals.

During the preparation from whole blood platelets and bacteria are concentrated in the same buffy coat-layer resulting in a higher initial bacterial number in platelets than in red cells. Platelets are stored at 24°C under agitation supporting growth of a great number of bacteria with high multiplication-rates at human body temperature (mesophilics). Mainly Gram-positive bacteria like staphylococci, coryne bacteria, streptococci and bacillus species, originated from the donor skin are seen. But also Gram-negative bacteria are described [27]. As sepsis is more frequently associated with platelets stored for longer periods, the acceptable storage period was reduced from 7 to 5 days [28].

Detection-techniques

Direct staining (Gram, acridine orange) and detection of pH and glucose-level has been evoked prior to issue of the blood-products. However these techniques can only detect numbers above 10^6 colony-forming units. Molecular biology (like polymerase chain reaction) is sensitive and can give quicker results but is still time consuming and the probes used limit the bacteria that can be detected.

Culturing has a sufficient sensitivity. Automated culturing devices can speed up logistics but about 24–48 hours are needed to detect most pathogenic bacteria [29,30]. The sensitivity is about 97% and specificity 98% (sampling errors can give false negative results [2]). Due to the composition of culturing media bacteria will better multiply in the culturing system than in the blood products themselves. Therefore even short-term bacterial culture is effective in reduction of platelet contamination and associated sepsis [12]. Red cells were contaminated with the same bacteria but less frequently than the platelets of the corresponding donation No contamination was detected in red cells of corresponding platelets with negative cultures [7]. In Sweden, Denmark and The Netherlands shelf life of cultured platelets are extended up to 7 days [7,31,32]. Platelets are issued as "negative to date" after a quarantine period of 48 hours. An additional positive economical benefit is obtained by decrease in outdated concentrates. In Belgium most transfusion centers are culturing all pooled platelets, but storage time is not extended [33]. In Germany 0.4 × the square root of total number of prepared blood products has to be screened [34].

Future actions

Zero contamination could be reached by inactivation of all microorganisms using psoralens and UVA light, but this technique will not be at hand before complete safety of these alkylating agents is established. For the mean time actions possible to reduce the incidence rate of TTI includes: improving the phlebotomy antisepsis when collecting the blood from the donor, discarding the first 10-15 ml of blood drawn from the donor, leukocyte reduction after 6–8 hours. The culture methodologies have to be standardized, including culturing of all platelet concentrates, and issue as negative to date. Pooled platelets could be used as indicator product for whole blood donation. Extension of shelf live of platelets can improve logistics and cut down costs.

References:

1. Morrow, JF, Braine HG et al: Septic reactions to platelet transfusion, a persistent problem. JAMA 1991; 266:555-58.
2. Blajchman MA, Ali AM et al: Bacteria in de blood supply: an overlooked issue in transfusion medicine. Blood safety: current challenges, AABB, 1992:213-28.
3. Noel L. Transfusion related bacterial sepsis as seen by the French hemovigilance. Presentation on Symposium on the non-sterility of blood and blood components, Luxembourg, September 4-6, 1996.
4. MMWR (Morbidity and Mortality Weekly Report). Editorial note, June 1997;46:554-55.
5. Barbara JAJ, McDonald et al: Bacteria in blood: they haven't gone away. Interface, lecture, 1998.
6. Korte, D de, Welle F et al: Determination of the degree of bacterial contamination of whole blood collections using Bact/Alert. Abstract, VI Regional ISBT Jerusalem, 1999.
7. Laan E, Tros C et al: Improving the safety and shelf life of leuko-depleted platelet concentrates by automated bacterial screening. Vox Sang 74S, abstract 1178, ISBT Oslo, Jun 27 – July 2, 1998.
8. Alvarez FE, Rogge KJ: Bacterial contamination of cellular blood components, a retrospective review at a large cancer center. Annals Clin Lab Science 1995; 25: 283-90.
9. Chiu EKW, Yuen KY: A prospective study of symptomatic bacteremia following platelet transfusion and of its management. Transfusion 1994;34: 950-54.

10. Gong J, Högman CF: Transfusion-associated Serratia marcescens infection: studies of the mechanism of action. Transfusion, 1993;33:802-08.
11. Klein, H.G, Dodd R.Y et al: Current status of microbial contamination of blood components summary of a conference. Transfusion 1997:37:95-101
12. Liu HW, Yuen KY et al: Reduction of platelet transfusion associated sepsis by short-term bacterial culture. Vox Sang 1999;77:1-5.
13. Sazama K: Bacteria in blood for transfusion, a review. Arch Pathol Lab Med, 1994;118:350-65.
14. Threlkeld MG, Cobbs CG et al: Infectious disorders of prosthetic valves and intravascular devices. In: Principles and practice of infectious diseases; Mandell, Douglas and Bennett, Churchill Livingstone Inc. 1995.
15. Perez P.L. Salmi R, et al: Determinants of transfusion-associated bacterial contamination: results of the French Bacthem Case-Control Study. Transfusion, 2001;41:862-72.
16. Gibson T, Norris W et al: Skin fragments removed by injection needles. Lancet, November 1958;983-85.
17. Blajchman MA: Bacterial contamination and proliferation during the storage of cellular blood products. Vox Sanguinis 1998;74(suppl 2):155-59.
18. Olthuis H, Puylaert C: Methods for removal of contaminating bacteria during vena puncture. Poster abstract 13, ISBT 1995 Venice.
19. Korte, D. de, Marcelis, J.H. et al: Reduction of the degree of bacterial contamination for whole blood collections. Abstract submitted AABB November 2000.
20. Bruneau C, Perez P, et al. Efficacy of a new collection procedure for preventing bacterial contamination of whole-blood donations. Transfusion: 2001;41:74-78.
21. Ness PM, Perkins HA et al: Transient bacteremia after dental procedures and other minor manipulations. Transfusion, 1980;20:82-85.
22. McQuiston, J.H, Childs, J.E. et al. Transmission of tick-borne agents of disease by blood transfusion: A review of known and potential risks in the United States. Transfusion 2000; 40: 274–84.
23. Pietersz RN, Reesink HW et al: Prevention of Yersinia enterocolitica growth in red-blood-cell concentrates. Lancet, 1992;340:755-56.
24. Högman CF, Gong J: White cells protect donor blood against bacterial contamination. Transfusion, 1991;31:620-26.
25. Gong J, Rawal BD et al: Complement killing of Yersinia enterocolitica and retention of the bacteria by leukocyte removal filters. Vox Sang 1994;66: 166-70.
26. Heltberg, O. Skov F, et al. Nosocomial epidemic of Serratia marcescens septicemia ascribed to contaminated blood transfusion bags. Transfusion 1993; 33:221-27.
27. Wagner SJ, Friedman LI, Dodd RY: Transfusion-associated bacterial sepsis. Clin Mircobiol Reviews 1994:290-302.
28. Anderson KC, Lew MA. Transfusion-related sepsis after prolonged platelet storage. Am J Med 1986;81:405-11.
29. Thorpe TC, Wilson ML et al: BacT/Alert: an automated colorimetric microbial detection system. J Clin Microbiology 1990;28:1608-12.

30. Brecher M.E., Norman Means N. Evaluation of an automated culture system for detecting bacterial contamination of platelets: An analysis with 15 contaminating organisms. Transfusion 2001;41:477-82.
31. Björk P: Bacterial screening of platelet concentrates–clinical experiences and economical consequences. Presentation on Symposium on the non-sterility of blood and blood components, Luxembourg, September 4-6, 1996
32. Øllgaard M, Albjerg I: Monitoring of bacterial growth in platelet concentrates–one year's experience with the BactAlert system. Vox Sang 74S, abstract 1126, ISBT Oslo, June 27–July 2, 1998.
33. Vandekerckhove B, van Vooren M. abstract VI ISBT Regional congress Jerusalem 2000.
34. Bundesgesundheitsblatt Gesundheitsforschung Gesundheitsschutz, 1999;42: 366.

PARASITES TRANSMITTED BY BLOOD TRANSFUSION

L.M. Kortbeek and E. Pinelli[1]

Introduction

Transmission of parasites by blood transfusion is considered to be an important issue especially with regard to global travel and land development that can alter the habitats of disease carrying insects and animals [1]. Different to viruses and bacteria, parasites have complicated life cycles that include different parasitic stages invading various tissues and in most cases an intermediate host is involved. Human parasitic infections are often asymptomatic or can develop into chronic diseases. This is probably one of the reasons why less attention has been given to infection with these pathogens. However, acute disease and major complication due to infection with parasites are commonly observed in immuno-compromised patients including, cancer, transplantation and HIV patients. Others that are also at risk in developing disease are less immuno-competent persons including children, elderly, undernourished and those suffering from other diseases at the time of infection.

This paper will review the protozoa (Table 1) that could represent a potential threat to the safety of blood supplies. The microbiology, epidemiology, clinical disease, diagnostics, treatment and transfusion acquired infections for several protozoan parasites are described.

Table 1. Parasitic diseases and the causative agents

Blood transmitted parasitic diseases	**Micro-organism**
Malaria	*Plasmodium spp.*
Babesiosis	*Babesia microti, B. divergens*
Toxoplasmosis	*Toxoplasma gondii*
Leishmaniasis	*Leishmania spp.*
Chagas disease	*Trypanosoma cruzi*

1. Diagnostic Laboratory for Infectious Diseases and Perinatal Screening, National Institute of Public Health and the Environment, Bilthoven, NL.

Malaria

Introduction

Malaria is by far the world's most important tropical parasitic disease. It is a public health problem today in more than 90 countries and has a worldwide prevalence of 300-500 million clinical cases each year with a mortality that is estimated to be over 1 million deaths each year. Malaria is transmitted by the bite of mosquitoes. The number and type of Anophiline mosquitoes in a given area determine the extent of transmission.

Microbiology and epidemiology

Malaria is caused by four different parasites of the same genus, Plasmodium vivax, Plasmodium ovale, Plasmodium malariae and Plasmodium falciparum. They cause different diseases, of which the most serious is malignant malaria or malaria tropica, brought on by Plasmodium falciparum. Plasmodium is a protozoan that invades during the asexual stage of its life cycle the red blood cells. The vector is a mosquito, Anopheles, of which there are many different species able to transmit malaria. The efficiency of transmission of malaria by the vector depends on the Anopheles subspecies.

Plasmodium falciparum is the most prevalent species in the tropics and subtropics. Plasmodium vivax is common in temperate zones but has been successfully eradicated in the USA and Western Europe. Plasmodium ovale is mostly found in tropical Africa and Plasmodium malariae occurs in tropical Africa and Southeast Asia [2,3]. In Africa, Asia and Latin America there is an increase in drug resistance of Plasmodium falciparum, and therefore a growing number of patients suffer from infections due to a multi-resistant P. falciparum strain. Chloroquine-resistant strains of P.vivax have been reported in Irian Jaya, Indonesia, and this problem seems to be spreading in Asia [4]. The life cycle is fairly complicated, with a sexual stage in the mosquito and an asexual stage in humans. The infection starts with a bite of the female Anopheles that injects the parasites into the bloodstream during a blood meal. The parasites invade the liver where they multiply during a few days to weeks. After this period they burst out of the hepatocytes and infect the red blood cells. They divide asexually in these red blood cells that burst every 2 or 3 days, thus causing the typical malaria attacks of fever. The mosquitoes are infected after taking a blood meal on an infected patient, ingesting the infected red blood cells with gametocytes. In the liver of Plasmodium vivax and Plasmodium ovale patients infected hepatocytes harbor dormant stages that can reactivate years after the primary infection. There is no liver stage in P. falciparum or P. malariae but as long as the asexual stages remain in the circulating blood the infection can be transmitted by transfusion. In Plasmodium malariae this can be as long as 40 years [3-5].

Most cases in the USA are import cases by people traveling to endemic areas. In 1997 P.vivax caused almost half of the reported cases (48.9%). P. falciparum was identified in 36.7% of the cases whereas P. ovale and P. malariae were detected only in 3.1% and 2.0% respectively. The time interval between the day of arrival from an endemic area and the occurrence of disease differ between the Plasmodium species. For P. vivax infected patients more than 50% of the cases develop symptoms later than 90 days after arrival. Ninety-five percent of the patients with P. falciparum will have symptoms within 90 days [6], and of these patients 88% will have symptoms within one month.

In Europe most (80%) of imported cases origin from Africa and in 70% P. falciparum is detected. However, in recent years a dramatically re-emergence of malaria occurred, due to political, social and economic reasons (Table 2).

Table 2: Number of autochthonous malaria cases in Europe in 1990 and 1999 (MacArthur 2001 [7])

Country	1990	1999
Armenia	0	329
Azerbaijan	24	2,311
Georgia	0	35
Greece	0	1
Kazakhstan	0	1
Russia fed.	7	77
Tajikistan	175	13,491
Turkey	8,675	20,905
Turkmenistan	0	10
Uzbekistan	3	7

Clinical symptoms and treatment

Malaria tropica (caused by Plasmodium falciparum) may exhibit quite a varied clinical picture, including fever, chills, sweating, cough and diarrhea up to shock, coma and death. The fatality rate among cases of untreated children and non-immune adults exceeds 10%. Malaria is particularly dangerous during pregnancy. It causes severe anemia, and is a major factor contributing to maternal deaths in endemic areas.

Malaria tertiana (caused by P. vivax and P. ovale) and malaria quartana (caused by P. malariae) are generally not life threatening, except in the very young, very old and immuno-compromised patient. Typical are the periods of fever, shaking chills, headache and nausea, ending in profuse sweating, alternating with a period free of symptoms.

The treatment of malaria depends on the species, drug resistance and severity of infection. In sensitive cases oral Chloroquine can be administered; in severe cases quinine IV can be given and in some infections with a high parasitaemia a massive blood-exchange transfusion can be necessary. The prognosis depends on the parasitaemia, involvement of the brain and the timely recognition of the disease. In the USA in 1997 six deaths were reported attributed to malaria [6]. In Europe 680 people died of malaria in the period 1989-1999 [7].

Diagnosis

Diagnosis is made by identification of the parasite by direct detection in a thick or thin blood film. Since a single examination of blood does not rule out the diagnosis, repeated examinations within 36 hours are required. The parasites can be seen in Giemsa stained blood smears but also other stains can be used (Wright's stain, Fields stain). Recently new techniques have been developed to demonstrate the parasites in a sensitive way, like Quantitative Buffy Coat (QBC) tubes for micro-hematocrit centrifugation, and dipsticks for antigen detection. Confirmation of these tests by tick and thin blood films are still recommended to confirm the identification of the species causing the infection. Differentiation between the species can be difficult due to minimal morphological differences.

Serology can be used to detect antibodies in cases of possible transfusion transmitted infection. The donor can be parasitologically negative (no parasites detectable) but antibodies can indicate that there has been an infection in the past. Malaria antibody detection can also be a valuable tool in the prevention of transfusion transmitted malaria in countries with a high proportion of donors with travel exposure to malaria [8].

There are molecular methods (PCR) available that have proved to be valuable for detection in a sensitive and rapid way. This has been used for follow-up studies of drug treatment and for typing different species [2].

Transfusion acquired infections

In the United States of America guidelines of the Food and Drug Administration and the American Association of Blood Banks have been implemented since 1994. According to these guidelines all travelers to malaria endemic areas should be deferred as a donor, and those who have been resident in a malaria endemic country or who report a history of malaria during three years [5, 9]. In a systematic review of all cases of transfusion transmitted malaria reported to the Centers for Disease Control and Prevention (CDC) from 1963 through 1999 with information about the implicated blood donors from the National Malaria Surveillance System 93 cases of transfusion transmitted malaria were reported in 28 states. Of these cases 33 (35%) were due to P. falciparum, 25 (27%) were due to P. vivax, 25 (27%) were due to P. malariae, 5 (5%) were due to P. ovale, 3 (3%) were mixed infections, and 2 (2%) were due to unidentified species. The incidence of transfusion-transmitted malaria in the United States has decreased in the past three decades and now remains at a stable low level with only one reported case per year. To determine whether donors should have been excluded from donating blood, the reviewers compared the characteristics of the donors with the exclusion guidelines of the Food and Drug Administration and the American Association of Blood Banks. Among those for whom complete information was available, 37 of 60 donors (62%) would have been excluded from donating according to current guidelines (in place since 1994), and 30 of 48 donors (63%) should have been excluded under the guidelines in place at the time of donation. The conclusion of the authors is that careful screening of donors according to the recommended exclusion guidelines remains the best way to prevent transfusion transmitted malaria [5,9].

In Europe only few reported cases of transfusion transmitted malaria can be found in recent literature. In the United Kingdom and Ireland there was 1 fatal case of transfusion transmitted malaria reported in the period October 1996 to September 1998 [10].

Babesiosis

Introduction

Babesiosis in an infection with a malaria-like protozoa that can be fatal in patients who do not have a spleen. Until some 30 years ago it was considered to be a veterinary problem, especially of cattle and sheep. However, since 1957 a fatal illness in splenectomized humans has been described. The parasite is transmitted by the bite of ticks.

Microbiology and epidemiology

There are different Babesia species found in humans. In the USA Babesia microti is the most prevalent species, although two other species have been described in humans. The WA type Babesia (in Washington: WA-1t/m3) causes a microti-like illness and the MO1 type Babesia (in the state Missouri MO-1) causing the more severe divergens-like illness [2,11-13]. In the USA the geographical distribution is related to the distribution of the most important vector, the tick Ixodes scapularis (formerly called Ixodes dammini) [14].

In Europe human infections caused by Babesia divergens have been reported from France, Ireland, Scotland, Spain, Sweden, Russia and Yugoslavia [15]. However recent studies in Spain, Poland and Slovenia using molecular techniques have reported the presence of B. microti in ticks in Europe [16]. The vector in Europe is the tick Ixodes ricinus. Recently a microti like Babesia and its vector Ixodes persulcatus have been reported in Japan (Saito-Ito2000). Babesia microti is transmitted primarily during the summer months by the bite of nymph or adult Ixodes ticks [14]. When the tick takes a blood meal, the infective stages are introduced into the human host and infect the red blood cells. The parasites resemble the early stages of malarial parasites [2]. Babesia can only be transmitted when the tick is allowed to stay on the patient for at least 36 hours. The incubation period is variable from 1 to 8 weeks.

Clinical symptoms and treatment

The clinical presentation of an infection with Babesia microti includes fever, hemolytic anemia, myalgia, joint pains and fatigue, lasting several days to months. Infection with Babesia divergens are more likely to be severe, with symptoms of hemoglobinuria like "red water"(red urine) and jaundice. The mortality in splenectomized patients is high.

The currently recommended treatment of symptomatic cases of Babesia microti is quinine plus clindamycin. In Babesia divergens infections a massive blood-exchange transfusion can be necessary, followed immediately by intravenous clindamycin (3-4 times daily) and oral quinine (600 mg base, 3 times daily) [11,14,15].

Diagnosis

Diagnosis in made by identification of the parasite by direct detection in a thick or thin blood film. The intra-erythrocytic organisms can be seen in Giemsa stained blood smears. The parasites are small (1-3 μm), pear shaped and can sometimes be seen as tetrads (Maltese cross) within the erythrocytes. Differentiation with P. falciparum can be difficult. This standard diagnostic technique for human infections has been complemented with serology and PCR [8]. Serology can also be useful for epidemiological studies. In the USA an immunofluorescence test (IFAT) is available but the cross-reactions between the strains is limited.

Transfusion acquired infections

In the U.S.A. 26 cases of Babesia infections acquired by blood transfusion have been reported. In seroprevalence studies, donor exposure rates of 3% or more in endemic areas have been reported. One of the proposed preventive measures is the exclusion of donors with high exposure risk. A problem with regard to blood transfusions is the asymptomatic patients. The proportion of asymptomatic infections is not known. However, in Japan an infection with a Babesia microti-like parasite from an asymptomatic donor has been reported [17]. In Europe, to our knowledge, no transfusion related cases have been reported.

Toxoplasmosis

Introduction

In Europe Toxoplasmosis is one of the most common parasitic diseases in man. Human infection with Toxoplasma gondii can be acquired congenitally or postnatally.

Microbiology and epidemiology

Toxoplasma gondii is a small, obligatory intracellular, protozoa with two different stages in man: trofozoite and bradyzoite. The trofozoite is the active form that divides asexually in all kind of cells. The bradyzoite is the inactive stage, lying in a tissue cyst in the different organs without any host reactivity around these cysts. The definitive host of Toxoplasma gondii is the cat. Oocysts are excreted by cats and can survive in the environment for a long period. Infection can occur by ingestion of oocysts in contaminated soil after working in the garden or eating vegetables or by ingestion of tissue cysts of intermediate hosts, when eating inadequately cooked or raw meat or by transmission of tissue cysts by organ transplantation. Furthermore, vertical transmission in pregnancy can result in congenital infection [2,19]. Recently the results of European risk factor studies in pregnant women show that the most important risk factor is consuming undercooked or raw meat [20-22].

Seroprevalence rates vary in the different countries between 8-11% in the UK and Norway and 58% in France [23].

Clinical symptoms and treatment

Toxoplasma infections can have different courses: The acute acquired infection (primary infection), the latent infection and reactivation. Re-activations of the latent infection occur, when tissue cysts burst and the immune system will be challenged. If the patient is immuno-suppressed the infection can have a serious outcome.

Most postnatally acquired infections are asymptomatic or present only with flu-like symptoms. In a minority of cases the infection is symptomatic. Although lymphadenopathy is the most common symptom, recurrent eye-disease can also be one of the symptoms [24-26]. Most infections will become latent infections within weeks or months, resulting in a persisting immunity. Furthermore, an infection during pregnancy can lead to severely affected children with retinochoroidal lesions, hydrocephalus and mental problems [19,27]. However, most children will be asymptomatic at birth. Ten to twenty% of all congenitally infected children have manifest disease. Long term follow-up showed that 80% of untreated infected children will develop ocular disease [28-30].

Treatment is usually not necessary in acquired infections because it is a self-limiting disease. Only for immuno-compromised patients and for congenital infected children, treatment is required.

Diagnosis

The methods used for the diagnosis of toxoplasmosis depend on the stage of infection. To diagnose an active, primary, infection the detection of IgM or IgA antibodies against Toxoplasma, together with the dynamics of IgG antibodies (rising titers) can give an indication. During pregnancy the detection of parasitic DNA in amniotic fluid can indicate transmission of the parasite from mother to fetus. This technique has almost replaced other techniques like culturing the amniotic fluid in mice or tissue cultures [31,32].To detect a latent infection with Toxoplasma detecting IgG antibodies will do. Diagnosis of reactivation of the infection can be difficult because the lack of good indicators. CT scans, rising titers and examination of spinal fluid by PCR can be of help.

Transfusion acquired infections

There are only a few documented cases of transfusion acquired Toxoplasmosis. Most of them are in old literature and the blood product involved is leukocyte concentrate [27]. The time period in which parasites can be found in the peripheral blood is short, probably only a few weeks. The immune response becomes detectable after 2 to 4 weeks. The risk that a healthy donor is parasitemic, is low. This is different in immuno-suppressed patients but they are not likely to be donors. Due to the relative low risk for recipients for acquiring Toxoplasma it seems unnecessary to establish routinely screening procedures in all blood donations. And if toxoplasmosis is considered to be a risk it is debatable whether sero-positive of sero-negative donors should be preferred. A sero-negative donor can still seroconvert and be parasitemic. A seropositive healthy donor is usually not parasitemic.

Leishmaniasis

Introduction

Leishmaniasis is a disease with different clinical manifestations caused by protozoan parasites of the genus Leishmania. The genus consists of different species that are epidemiologically diverse and complex. Leishmania spp. are obligate intracellular pathogens that are engulfed by macrophages of the mammalian host. These parasites are transmitted by the bite of infected sand flies. Depending on the species involved, infection with Leishmania spp. can result in cutaneous, muco-cutaneous or visceral leishmaniasis.

Microbiology and epidemiology

Visceral leishmaniasis is caused in China, India, the Middle East and Africa by L. donovani and in North Africa and the Mediterranean region by L. infantum. In Latin America the infectious agent is L. chagasi.

The infectious agents of cutaneous leishmaniasis in the Old World are Leishmania tropica, L. major and L. aethiopica. In the New World the disease is caused by species of the L. braziliensis and L. mexicana complexes. Species of the L. braziliensis complex are most likely to produce muco-cutaneous leishmaniasis that focally occur from Texas (USA) and Mexico to Central and South America [33].

The World Health Organization (WHO) estimates 1.5 million cases of cutaneous leishmaniasis and 500,000 clinical cases of visceral leishmaniasis occur every year in 82 countries. Estimates indicate that there are more that 350 million people at risk of acquiring leishmaniasis with 12 million currently infected (World Health Organization WHO/ LEISH/200.42) [34]. The risk factors for acquiring leishmaniasis have been reported to be increasing worldwide [35].

Clinical symptoms and treatment

Skin ulcers that may poorly heal, often leaving scars, characterize cutaneous leishmaniasis. Infected macrophages are found in these skin lesions. Muco-cutaneous leishmaniasis occurs when the cutaneous lesions spread to mucosal membranes of the mouth, nose and pharynx, giving rise to highly disfiguring swellings and destruction of the tissue. Fever, coughing diarrhea, anemia, wasting and enlargement of the liver and spleen characterize the visceral form, which is fatal unless treated. Although, the different clinical manifestations depend primarily on the species of Leishmania causing infection, it can also depend on the general state of health, age and genetic make-up of the host [36]. Simple lesions of cutaneous leishmaniasis will generally heal spontaneously, but it can take a year or more. Treatment options include cryo-therapy, heat, surgical excision of the lesion and chemotherapy. Standard therapy consists of injections with antimonial compounds such as Pentostam or Glucantime. The disadvantages of using antimonial compounds are the side effects. Amphotericin B and imidazoles have been used as successful alternatives to antimonial therapy [37].

Diagnosis

Diagnosis of leishmaniasis depends on the identification of the intracellular form of the parasite (amastigote) in tissues. The material to be analyzed include skin, bone marrow, spleen, liver and lymph node biopsies, scrapings or aspirates. Microscopical observation of Giemsa stained slides is the direct way of identifying amastigotes. The extracellular form of the parasites (promastigote) can also be identified after culture of the material taken from the patient. Monoclonal antibodies and DNA probes are also used to detect infections. PCR is a reliable diagnostics test with higher sensitivity than routine smears and culture. Blood samples can also be used as material for diagnostic of leishmaniasis using PCR. This technique allows the identification of the Leishmania species involved [38-40]. Serology can be used for diagnosis of visceral leishmaniasis. The techniques used for analysis include IFA (immunofluorescence), ELISA, DAT (direct agglutination test) and Western Blots. For cutaneous leishmaniasis serological tests are not very useful since patients with this clinical manifestation have very low if any antibody titers.

Transfusion acquired infections

Although, reports of transfusion transmitted leishmaniasis have been mainly anecdotal, and in no case was the donor identified, the circulation of L. infantum in the blood of healthy sero-positive individuals has been shown by Le Fichoux et al. in an area of endemicity in southern France. The authors suggest the leucodepletion of the blood to be used for transfusions [41]. Leishmania amastigotes have also been detected in the peripheral blood smears of Indian kala-azar patients mostly during the night [42].
The identification of Leishmania-infected blood products has been identified for donors from the Operation Desert Storm. The blood components that have been implicated are whole blood, packed red blood cells, platelet concentrate, and frozen-deglycerolized red blood cells, but not fresh frozen plasma [43].

Further evidence on transmission of Leishmania spp. through blood is represented by studies showing the existence of a leishmaniasis outbreak among intravenous drug users in northeast Spain [44].

Trypanosomiasis

Introduction

Trypanosomes are hemoflagellates that live in the blood and tissues of their human hosts. African trypanosomiasis or sleeping sickness is caused by parasites of the Trypanosoma brucei complex. These protozoan parasites are transmitted to the mammalian host by the bite of the tsetse fly. There are few reports on transfusion transmitted African trypanosomiasis [46].

American Trypanosomiasis or Chagas disease is caused by T. cruzi and T. rangeli. The disease is transmitted to humans through the bite wound caused by reduviid bugs. The second most important way of acquiring Chagas disease is by blood transfusion.

Microbiology and epidemiology

In America, infections with T. rangeli are asymptomatic, with no evidence of pathology. Infections with T. cruzi however, can cause considerable morbidity and mortality. These parasites can migrate from blood to different tissues invading cells of the heart, esophagus and colon. Chagas disease is one of the major problems in Latin American countries. It is estimated that 100 million persons are at risk of infection. There are 16 million to 18 million that are actually infected. Approximately 50,000 deaths per year are caused by infection with T. cruzi. Transmission of this parasite can also take place through blood transfusions, organ transplantation and placental transfer [45].

Clinical symptoms and treatment

The clinical symptoms for Chagas disease can be separated in initial, acute, indeterminate and chronic stages. The initial stage usually passes unnoticed but there may be an inflamed swelling or chagoma at the site of entry of the trypanosomes. Symptoms during the acute stage are fever, hepato-splenomegaly, myalgia, lymphadenopathy, myocarditis, keratitis and subcutaneous edemas on the face legs and feet.

Several drugs have been tried for the treatment of patients with Chagas disease, including those used for African trypanosomiasis and leishmaniasis. Currently available drugs (nitrofurans and nitroimidazoles) are active in acute or short-term chronic infections, but have very low antiparasitic activity against the prevalent chronic form of the disease, and toxic side-effects are frequently encountered. The nitroimidazole benznidazole has also shown significant activity in the treatment of reactivated Trypanosoma cruzi infections in patients with acquired immune deficiency syndrome and in other immunosuppressed patients with underlying chronic Chagas disease [47].

Diagnosis

Physical findings and clinical history is very important in establishing the diagnosis. Exposure to the vectors, residence in or travel to areas where the disease is endemic, or recent blood transfusion in these areas, are important aspects to consider. Definite diagnosis depends on demonstrations of the parasites in blood, amastigote stages in tissues or positive serological reactions. The serological tests used for the diagnosis of Chagas disease include complement fixation, immunofluorescence and ELISA.

These parasites can also be detected using molecular tools including PCR. The advantage of this technique is that it is very sensitive and specific, compared to the serological tests available.

Transfusion acquired infections

Transmission of Chagas disease by blood transfusions is considered the second most common way of acquiring this infection [48]. Infection rates among blood recipients vary from 1.4% to 18% in Argentinia, Brazil, and Chile and can be up to 48% in Bolivia [49]. Only Venezuela and Honduras screened 100% the donors in 1993 (Table 3). The absolute number of T. cruzi transfusion transmitted infections varied in 1993/1994 from 7 in Honduras to 875 in Colombia

Table 3. Serology for Trypanosoma cruzi in blood donors in 1993 (Schmunis, 1999 [49])

Country	No. of donors	Screening coverage (% of donors with serology)	Prevalence (00)
Bolivia	37,948	29.4	14.81
Chile	217,312	76.7	1.20
Colombia	352,316	1.4	1.20
El Salvador	48,048	42.5	1.47
Ecuador (1994)	98,473	51.0	0.20
Guatemala	45,426	75.0	1.40
Honduras	27,885	100.0	1.24
Nicaragua	46,001	58.4	0.24
Paraguay (1994)	32,893	95.4	5.30
Venezuela	203,316	100.0	1.32

Table 4. Trypanosoma cruzi transfusion transmitted infection* (Schmunis, 1999 [49])

Country	Probability of receiving an infected transfusion (x0000)†	Probability of getting a transfusion transmitted infection (x0000)†	Absolute no. of transfusion transmitted infections	Ratio infections/ donations
Bolivia	1096.38	219.28	832	1:46
Chile	29.36	5.87	236	1:92
Colombia	124.24	24.85	875	1:403
Ecuador	10.29	2.06	20	1:4,924
El Salvador	88.75	17.75	85	1:565
Guatemala	36.75	7.35	33	1:1,377
Honduras	13.02	2.60	7	1:3,984
Nicaragua	10.48	2.10	10	1:4,600
Paraguay	62.37	12.47	41	1:802
Venezuela	13.86	2.77	57	1:3,584

* Data from 1993, except for Ecuador and Paraguay that were 1994;
† Probability for 10,000 transfusions.
Residual infection only as screening coverage is 100%.

(Table 4). Few years later, in 1997 also Argentina, Brazil, Colombia, El Salvador, Paraguay and Uruguay carried out 100% screening of the donors reducing this way the number of T. cruzi transfusion transmitted infections [48]. a: data from 1993, except for Ecuador and Paraguay that were 1994; b: probability for 10,000 transfusions. c: residual infection only as screening coverage is 100%.

Concluding remarks

Several aspects must be considered in relation to blood transfusion transmitted parasitic diseases in countries where these infections are not endemic. It is important to be aware of

- The epidemiology of the relevant parasitic diseases;
- The donors' country of origin;
- Changes in the composition of the country's population and therefore of the donor's population due to immigration and travelling. These changes in the population's composition is also affected by the frequent back and forth travelling of the second (or more) generation of immigrants to their country of origin where they will be exposed to endemic infections;
- Certain parasitic infections are not only common in tropical countries but are also endemic in "Western" countries such as Babesia in USA and Leishmania spp. in France;
- Screening donors with serological test can reveal an infection but a negative test does not exclude an infection;
- Asymptomatic patients represent a major risk for the transmission of parasites by blood transfusion;
- The parasites here descibed are small organisms (1-20 μm) that are present either in red blood cells, leucocytes or free living in blood. The procedure used to generate safe blood products should take this into account.

References

1. Chamberland ME. Emerging Infectious Agents: Do They Pose a Risk to the Safety of Transfused Blood and Blood Products? Clin.Infect.Dis. 2002;34: 797-805.
2. Malaria and babesia. Garcia LS, Bruckner DA III, ASM. Diagnostic Medical Parasitology. Washington DC, 1997:135-66. Ref Type: Serial (Book, Monograph).
3. Malaria. Chin J. 17, APHA. Control of communicable diseases. Washington DC. 2002:310-23. Ref Type: Serial (Book, Monograph).
4. Baird JK, Wiady I, Fryauff DJ, et al. In Vivo Resistance to Chloroquine by Plasmodium Vivax and Plasmodium Falciparum at Nabire, Irian Jaya, Indonesia. Am J Trop Med Hyg 1997;56:627-31.
5. Mungai M, Tegtmeier G, Chamberland M, Parise M. Transfusion-Trans mitted Malaria in the United States From 1963 Through 1999. N Engl J Med 2001;344:1973-78.
6. MacArthur JR. Malaria Surveillance-United States, 1997. MMWR 50(SS01) 2001:25-44. Ref Type: Generic.
7. Sabatinelli G, Ejov M, Joergensen P. Malaria in the WHO European Region (1971-1999). Euro Surveill 2001;6:61-65.
8. Silvie O, Thellier M, Rosenheim M, et al. Potential Value of Plasmodium Falciparum-Associated Antigen and Antibody Detection for Screening of

Blood Donors to Prevent Transfusion- Transmitted Malaria. Transfusion 2002;42:357-62.
9. Dodd RY. Transmission of Parasites by Blood Transfusion. Vox Sang. 1998; 74 (Suppl 2):161-63.
10. Williamson LM, Lowe S, Love EM, et al. Serious Hazards of Transfusion (SHOT) Initiative: Analysis of the First Two Annual Reports. BMJ 1999; 319:16-19.
11. Herwaldt B, Persing DH, Precigout EA, et al. A Fatal Case of Babesiosis in Missouri: Identification of Another Piroplasm That Infects Humans. Ann Intern Med 1996;124:643-50.
12. Herwaldt BL, Springs FE, Roberts PP, et al. Babesiosis in Wisconsin: a Potentially Fatal Disease. Am J Trop Med Hyg 1995;53:146-51.
13. Herwaldt BL, Kjemtrup AM, Conrad PA, et al. Transfusion-Transmitted Babesiosis in Washington State: First Reported Case Caused by a WA1-Type Parasite. J Infect Dis 1997;175:1259-62.
14. Babesiosis. Chin J. APHA. Control of communicable diseases. Washington DC, 2000;17: 62-63. Ref Type: Serial (Book, Monograph).
15. Brasseur P and Gorenflot A. Human Babesiosis in Europe. Mem Inst Oswaldo Cruz 1992;87 (Suppl 3):131-32.
16. Duh D, Petrovec M, Avsic-Zupanc T. Diversity of Babesia Infecting European Sheep Ticks (Ixodes Ricinus). J Clin Microbiol 2001;39:3395-97.
17. Saito-Ito A, Tsuji M, Wei Q, et al. Transfusion-Acquired, Autochthonous Human Babesiosis in Japan: Isolation of Babesia Microti-Like Parasites With Hu-RBC-SCID Mice. J Clin Microbiol 2000;38:4511-16.
18. Kjemtrup AM and Conrad PA. Human Babesiosis: an Emerging Tick-Borne Disease. Int J Parasitol 2000;30:1323-37.
19. Gilbert RE. Epidemiology of infection in pregnant women. In: Peterson E, Ambroise-Thomas P. eds. Congenital toxoplasmosis: sientific background, clinical managment and control. Spronger-Verlag, Paris, France. 2000:237-49. Type: Serial (Book, Monograph).
20. Buffolano W, Gilbert RE, Holland FJ, Fratta D, Palumbo F, Ades AE. Risk Factors for Recent Toxoplasma Infection in Pregnant Women in Naples. Epidemiol Infect 1996;116:347-51.
21. Cook AJ, Gilbert RE, Buffolano W, et al. Sources of Toxoplasma Infection in Pregnant Women: European Multicentre Case-Control Study. European Research Network on Congenital Toxoplasmosis. BMJ 2000;321:142-47.
22. Kapperud G, Jenum PA, Stray-Pedersen B, Melby KK, Eskild A, Eng J. Risk Factors for Toxoplasma Gondii Infection in Pregnancy. Results of a Prospective Case-Control Study in Norway. Am J Epidemiol 1996;144:405-12.
23. Tenter AM, Heckeroth AR, Weiss LM. Toxoplasma Gondii: From Animals to Humans. Int J Parasitol 2000;30:1217-58.
24. Bosch-Driessen EH and Rothova A. Recurrent Ocular Disease in Postnatally Acquired Toxoplasmosis. Am J Ophthalmol 1999;128:421-25.
25. Bosch-Driessen LE, Berendschot TT, Ongkosuwito JV, Rothova A. Ocular Toxoplasmosis: Clinical Features and Prognosis of 154 Patients. Ophthalmology 2002;109:869-78.

26. Silveira C, Belfort R Jr, Muccioli C, et al. A Follow-Up Study of Toxoplasma Gondii Infection in Southern Brazil. Am J Ophthalmol 2001;131: 351-54.
27. Remington JS, Desmonts G. Toxoplasmosis. In: Remington JS, Klein JO.. Infectious diseases of the fetus and newborn infant. WB Saunders Company 1983:143-263. Ref Type: Serial (Book, Monograph).
28. Koppe JG, Loewer-Sieger DH, Roever-Bonnet H. Results of 20-Year Follow-Up of Congenital Toxoplasmosis. Lancet 1986;1:254-56.
29. Koppe JG. Prevention of Congenital Toxoplasmosis. Ned TijdschrGeneeskd 1992;136:1501-04.
30. Koppe JG and Meenken C. Congenital Toxoplasmosis, Later Relapses and Treatment. Acta Paediatr 1999;88:586-88.
31. Kupferschmidt O, Kruger D, Held TK, Ellerbrok H, Siegert W, Janitschke K. Quantitative Detection of Toxoplasma Gondii DNA in Human Body Fluids by TaqMan Polymerase Chain Reaction. Clin Microbiol Infect 2001;7: 120-24.
32. Hitt JA and Filice GA. Detection of Toxoplasma Gondii Parasitemia by Gene Amplification, Cell Culture, and Mouse Inoculation. J Clin Microbiol 1992;30:3181-84.
33. Das P. Infectious Disease Surveillance Update. Lancet Infect Dis 2002;2: 203.
34. Choi CM and Lerner EA. Leishmaniasis As an Emerging Infection. J Investig Dermatol (Symp.Proc) 2001;6:175-82.
35. Desjeux P. Worldwide Increasing Risk Factors for Leishmaniasis. Med Microbiol Immunol (Berl) 2001;190:77-79.
36. Cunningham AC. Parasitic Adaptive Mechanisms in Infection by Leishmania. Exp Mol Pathol 2002;72:132-41.
37. Gangneux JP and Marty P. Treatment of Visceral Leishmaniasis: Efficacy and Limits of Miltefosine. Sante 2001;11:257-58.
38. Osman OF, Oskam L, Zijlstra EE, et al. Evaluation of PCR for Diagnosis of Visceral Leishmaniasis. J Clin Microbiol 1997;35:2454-57.
39. Osman OF, Oskam L, Kroon NC, et al. Use of PCR for Diagnosis of Post-Kala-Azar Dermal Leishmaniasis. J Clin Microbiol 1998;36:1621-24.
40. Schonian G, Schweynoch C, Zlateva K, et al. Identification and Determination of the Relationships of Species and Strains Within the Genus Leishmania Using Single Primers in the Polymerase Chain Reaction. Mol Biochem Parasitol 1996;77:19-29.
41. Le Fichoux Y, Quaranta JF, Aufeuvre JP, et al. Occurrence of Leishmania Infantum Parasitemia in Asymptomatic Blood Donors Living in an Area of Endemicity in Southern France. J Clin Microbiol 1999;37:1953-57.
42. Sharma MC, Gupta AK, Das VN, et al. Leishmania Donovani in Blood Smears of Asymptomatic Persons. Acta Trop 2000;76:195-96.
43. Grogl M, Daugirda JL, Hoover DL, Magill AJ, Berman JD. Survivability and Infectivity of Viscerotropic Leishmania Tropica From Operation Desert Storm Participants in Human Blood Products Maintained Under Blood Bank Conditions. Am J Trop Med Hyg 1993;49:308-15.

44. Morales MA, Chicharro C, Ares M, Canavate C, Barker DC, Alvar J. Molecular Tracking of Infections by Leishmania Infantum. Trans R Soc Trop Med Hyg 2001;95:104-07.
45. Prata A. Clinical and Epidemiological Aspects of Chagas Disease. Lancet Infect Dis 2001;1:92-100.
46. Wendel S. Current Concepts on Transmission of Bacteria and Parasites by Blood Components. Vox Sang 1994;67(Suppl 3):161-74.
47. Urbina JA. Specific Treatment of Chagas Disease: Current Status and New Developments. Curr Opin Infect Dis 2001;14:733-41.
48. Schmunis GA, Zicker F, Cruz JR, Cuchi P. Safety of Blood Supply for Infectious Diseases in Latin American Countries, 1994-1997. Am J Trop Med Hyg 2001;65:924-30.
49. Schmunis GA. Prevention of Transfusional Trypanosoma Cruzi Infection in Latin America. Mem Inst Oswaldo Cruz 1999;94(Suppl 1):93-101.

RION DISEASES AND BLOOD TRANSFUSION

Marc L.Turner[1]

Introduction

The transmissible spongiform encephalopathies (TSE) comprise a spectrum of diseases in animals and man. Scrapie was first described over 200 years ago and is endemic in sheep and goats throughout large parts of the world. There is no evidence, however, that it has ever transmitted to man. Chronic Wasting Disease is endemic in Rocky Mountain Elk and Mule Deer in the USA and again there is no direct good evidence that it is transmissible to man. Transmissible Mink Encephalopathy (TME) described in farmed mink in Wisconsin, may have been transmitted via contaminated food. Bovine Spongiform Encephalopathy (BSE) was first described in the United Kingdom in 1985. Infected cattle display characteristic clinical features in which they become hypersensitive, ataxic and difficult to handle, hence giving rise to the colloquial name "Mad Cow Disease". It is thought that the disease either arose spontaneously in cattle or was transmitted from scrapie infected sheep, and was thereafter propagated via rendered meat and bone meal products. More than 180,000 clinical cases of BSE have been described to date in the UK, and although the incidence of the disease continues to decline, 1,300 further cases were described in 2000. It is thought that up to another 750,000 cases of BSE could have entered the human food chain prior to the development of clinical disease. About 1,500 cases of BSE have been described in other European countries thus far. Natural and experimental transmission of BSE has occurred in up to twenty different species including domestic and exotic cats and exotic ungulates in British zoos.

Sporadic Creutzfeldt-Jakob Disease (CJD) was first described in 1922 and presents in a relatively elderly population (median age 68 years) with a rapidly progressive dementia leading to death over a period of around six months. The incidence of sporadic CJD is around one in a million on a worldwide basis with no evidence of a relationship with animal TSEs such as scrapie . Kuru was described in the Foré people of Papua New Guinea in the 1950s and presented a different clinical picture consisting of cerebellar ataxia and a more prolonged duration of clinical disease. The disease is thought to have been orally transmitted during cannibalistic funeral rights. The incidence of the disease has gradually diminished following the cessation of these practices in around 1960, however a handful of clinical cases of Kuru continue to

1. Clinical director, Scottish National Blood Transfusion Service, Edinburgh, UK.

present, highlighting the very prolonged incubation periods that can occur in some individuals with these diseases. Iatrogenic CJD can arise in one of two ways. Central nervous system transmission can occur via contaminated neurosurgical instruments or dura mater grafts and gives rise to a clinical picture similar to that seen in sporadic CJD after a short incubation period of around two years. In contrast, peripherally transmitted CJD due to parenteral administration of cadaveric pituitary growth or follicular stimulating hormones is clinically more similar to Kuru and has a median incubation period in the 13–15 year range.

Variant CJD was first described in 1996 [1] and thus far just over a hundred cases have been described, the vast majority in the United Kingdom with a further 6 in France and one each in Ireland, Hong Kong and Italy. The median age at presentation is around 29 years with a range from 12 to 74 years. The clinical presentation is one of psychiatric symptoms such as anxiety and depression, followed by development of sensory disturbance and ataxia leading to terminal dementia and death over a period of 6–24 months [2-4]. The clinical, epidemiological, neuropathological and experimental evidence all strongly support the thesis that variant CJD represents the same strain of disease as BSE, most likely transmitted through infected food products [5-11]. It remains unclear how many people may currently be incubating the disease. Estimates range from current numbers up to 140,000 clinical cases over the next few decades. Uncertainty arises due to our lack of knowledge about the efficiency of oral transmission of BSE to man and the possible median and range of incubation periods of variant CJD [12,13].

Finally there are a small number of cases of human TSE caused by mutations in the prion (PrP) gene which include familial CJD, Gerstmann Straussler-Scheinker Disease and Fatal Familial Insomnia.

The Pathophysiology of Disease

This is therefore a very interesting group of diseases which can arise spontaneously, are known to be transmissible and can also be genetically inherited. No DNA has thus far been shown to be transmitted with TSEs, yet a number of different disease strains have been described. It is thought that this group of diseases is caused by changes in the secondary structure of normal human prion protein (PrP^C). PrP^C is a 30–35 KD GPI-anchored glycoprotein with two N-linked glycosylation sites. About 40% of its secondary structure consists of alpha helices and about 3% beta pleated sheets. During the development of TSEs, PrP^C undergoes conformational transformation with an increase in the beta-pleated sheet up to around 40% of the molecule, mainly at the expense of the relatively unstructured membrane distal region. This leads to increased resistance due to normal degradation mechanisms and accumulation of amyloid plaques in affected tissues (termed PrP^{SC}). The pathogenesis remains unclear but it is thought that the initial template acts as a core around which further conformational change occurs. In the brains of affected animals PrP^{SC} accumulation leads to neuronal death and reactive astrogliosis resulting in classical spongiform change. Amyloid plaques consisting of PrP^{SC} are particularly florid in variant CJD [14].

TSEs do not appear to give rise to extra neural disease. However it is known that PrP^{C} itself is widely distributed in extra neural tissues. Work by ourselves and others has demonstrated that the amount of PrP^{C} in normal human peripheral blood is between 10 and 300 ng/ml with around 68% of this distributed in the plasma, 27% in the platelets, 3% in the leucocytes (predominantly the mononuclear cells) and 1%–2% in the erythrocytes [15,16] Whether abnormal PrP^{SC} will prove to be detectable in the peripheral blood remains unclear for reasons which will be discussed below. However, it is known that abnormal accumulation of PrP^{SC} does occur in the peripheral lymphoid tissue of patients with variant CJD, specifically in the follicular dendritic cells of the spleen, lymph nodes and gut associated lymphoid tissue [17]. In one individual, PrP^{SC} was found in an appendix specimen taken some eight months prior the development of clinical variant CJD [18]. This peripheral distribution of PrP^{SC} is a feature not seen in sporadic CJD, and raises the possibility that variant CJD poses a higher risk of transmission of infection from blood and lymphoid tissues than sporadic disease.

Assessing the level of risk

It is known from studies in experimental animal models that following parenteral challenge with experimental TSE strains, infectivity can be detected in peripheral lymphatic tissue from an early stage of infection, preceding the detection of infectivity in the nervous system and persisting throughout the incubation phase of the disease [19].

Considerable work has been undertaken in assessing the presence and level of infectivity in the peripheral blood of animals with various strains of TSE . No activity has ever been demonstrated in peripheral blood in natural scrapie in sheep and goats, naturally occurring transmissible mink encephalopathy or in natural or experimental BSE in cattle. However peripheral blood infectivity has been demonstrated in experimental scrapie and BSE in sheep and rodents and in an experimental strain of GSS disease in rodents, during both the clinical and incubation phases of disease [20]. The level of infectivity is however many orders of magnitude less than that seen in the brain, amounting to around 100 infectious units/ml during the clinical phase of disease and 5–10 infectious units/ml during the incubation period [21]. Brown has undertaken detailed studies of the distribution of blood infectivity in mice infected with the Fukuoka strain of GSS. He found a 3-4 fold higher level of infectivity in the buffy coat compared to plasma, and that plasma showed a 10 fold higher concentration of infectivity compared to various Cohn fractions [21,22]. Rhower has published similar findings in the 293K hamster model and has also demonstrated that 5-7 times more buffy coat is required to transmit disease by the intravenous route compared to the intracerebral route [23]. Transmission of BSE by intravenous transfusion of blood drawn from experimentally orally infected sheep during the incubation phase of disease has also been described [24].

In man, cerebral infectivity levels are in the order of 10^6 to 10^7 infectious units/mg, several orders of magnitude less than that seen in experimentally infected animals. There are 5 reports out of 37 cases studied reporting transmission of sporadic CJD from human peripheral blood drawn during the clinical phase of disease by intracerebral inoculation into rodents [25]. However there are methodological criticisms of these studies and Brown reports no transmission of sporadic CJD from human peripheral blood to primates by intracerebral inoculation. No transmission of variant CJD from human peripheral blood to rodents or primates has as yet been described though most of these experiments are still within relatively early phases.

In the clinical setting there are 3 anecdotal case reports of patients developing sporadic CJD who have previously been exposed to blood components or products. However in none of these is there well substantiated evidence of transmission from an infected donor. Indeed a large number of epidemiological case control, look back and surveillance studies carried out over the last 20 years have shown no evidence of an increase risk of sporadic CJD in blood component or plasma product recipients. However some caution should be expressed in the interpretation of these observations, sporadic CJD remains a very rare disease and occasional cases of transmission could have been missed by these studies. In addition the prevalence of pre-clinical variant CJD may be much higher amongst the UK donor population, variant CJD represents a different strain of TSE and route to infection. Finally, there may not yet have been sufficient time for secondary infections to present clinically if they are occurring.

The risk of transmission of variant CJD by blood components and products therefore remains uncertain.

Strategies for risk containment

Donor selection

Within the United Kingdom there are no clear risk factor s predisposing to the development of variant CJD . Epidemiological the prevalence of variant CJD is proportionally higher in Scotland and the North of England (2.7 per million per annum) compared to the South of England and Wales (1 per million per annum) [26,27]. Occasional clusters are now becoming apparent such as that described in Queniborough in Leicestershire [28]. Elsewhere, many countries have taken steps to defer donors who have been resident in the United Kingdom. There is no evidence to inform the decision as to how long a period of residence represents a significant risk and donor exclusion criteria have been based on maximum tolerable donor loss. Most countries have adopted a cumulative 6 month period between 1980 and 1996 as a cut off.

There are some other groups of potentially high risk individuals who could be excluded from blood donation including those who themselves have received blood components or plasma products and those who have undergone surgery or other invasive medical procedures. However, the negative impact on blood supplies of implementation of many of these policies is likely to be significant and the reduction in the risk of variant CJD transmission uncertain.

Sourcing of blood components and plasma products from variant CJD -free countries

For countries with clinical cases of variant CJD, one option is to source blood components from variant CJD /BSE free countries. The UK already imports plasma for plasma product manufacturer from Europe and the United States. Though it is unlikely to be practical to source all red cell and platelet concentrates for the UK from out with the country, the sourcing of clinical plasma or cryoprecipitate may be feasible. Another option under consideration is selective sourcing of blood components for certain categories of (most vulnerable) recipients. Candidate groups include neonates and children born after 1996 on the grounds that these individuals are unlikely to have been exposed to BSE through the food chain and have longest potential life expectancy within which to manifest clinical disease.

Development of diagnostic / screening peripheral blood assays

Considerable work is ongoing into the development of diagnostic screening assays. Part of the problem is that there is no conventional immune response or detectable DNA associated with these diseases and so traditional serological and molecular biological approaches are not applicable. A number of non-specific makers of CNS damage which are currently under examination including 14-3-3 and S100 [29]. In addition decreased expression of erythroid differentiation related factor (EDRF) in the bone marrow and peripheral blood of scrapie infected sheep and rodents and of BSE infected cattle has recently been described [30]. This finding suggests that TSE infection may have a subtle impact on the peripheral haematopoietic and immune systems and that some hitherto unforeseen surrogate markers of disease may be available.

In terms of detection of PrP^{SC} in the peripheral blood, there are a number of issues surrounding specificity and sensitivity. The abnormal conformer could in principle be discriminated by monoclonal antibodies, but thus far only one such antibody has been described and this not widely available [31]. Other binding agents such as plasminogen have been described as demonstrating specificity to the abnormal conformer [32]. The strongest evidence suggests that physico-chemical methods of discrimination of PrP^{SC} such as insolubility in non-ionic surfactants, resistance to proteinase-K digestion and changes in epitope exposure due to chaotropic agents may be the best discriminators. However caution needs to be exercised in that these are often relative rather than absolute differences between the normal and abnormal isoforms of PrP. Sensitivity in PrP^{SC} detection is also a central issue. Assuming that the infectivity in human blood is between 10 and 100 IU/ml this translates to a physical detection limit of 1 pg/ml of PrP^{SC} [20] in the presence of 10-300 ng/ml of normal PrP^{C} [16]. A number of assays are currently under development including Western blot [33], competitive fluorescence capillary electrophoresis [34] and dissociation enhanced lanthanide fluorescence immunoassay [35] though none has as yet achieved the level of sensitivity likely to be required. Other important issues include the ratio of PrP^{SC} to infectivity, which may vary dependent on the strain of TSE, the animal species and the tissue of detection. Assay validation is likely to be problematic given the duration of incubation period of these diseases both in animals and man. Issues surrounding the development of standardised reagents and confirmatory testing strategies, applicability to large scale screening and the potential negative impact on the donor population of introduction of any screening strategy need to be addressed.

Blood component processing

Blood component processing has the potential to reduce infectivity. A number of countries have introduced universal leucocyte depletion predicated on the observation that in experimental systems in which infectivity is found in the peripheral blood, the highest concentrations are present in the buffy coat. Leucocyte depletion removes 3–4 $\log_{10}$ leucocytes with no evidence of differential removal of subsets or of significant fragmentation [36]. However whether this strategy is necessary or sufficient to reduce the risk of transmission of variant CJD remains uncertain. Certainly the data demonstrating that the majority of normal PrP^{C} is present in platelets and plasma goes some way to undermine confidence in the efficacy of this strategy. Further strategies could include washing of red cell and platelet concentrates, though the logistics involved in such a policy would be very substantial and although this would result in a significant reduction in PrP^{C} the potential impact on PrP^{SC}, which is largely cell associated, is less clear. The possibility of utilising absorption or affinity columns using either PrP specific monoclonal antibodies or other adhesive compounds has been suggested. However difficulties lie in the high ratio of PrP^{C} to PrP^{SC} in the peripheral blood and in the consequent removal of PrP expressing cells.

Prophylactic or therapeutic agents

A number of agents have shown inhibitory effects on PrP^{SC} accumulation in *in vitro* cell free or cell based systems and/or in *in vivo* experimental transmission models in rodents. Some of these such as porphyrins and phthalocyanines [37] may have potential to be added to blood components. Others, such as pentosan sulphate [38] and various immunosuppressive agents could be used to inhibit progression of disease in patients who are known to have received transfusion from an at risk patient or prove to be positive on a diagnostic or screening peripheral blood assay. Some such as anti-malarials and phenothiazenes may be of some value in patients who develop neurological disease [39].

Optimal use of blood

It is very clear that there is widespread variation in the use of blood components and products and there is an urgent need to implement clinical strategies to reduce blood usage both to manage the risk of unnecessary exposure to variant CJD infected blood and to reduce the overall demand on the blood supply at a time when significant blood donor loss may occur.

Major issues in policy making

The uncertainty surrounding the risk of transmission of variant CJD via blood transfusion has brought to the surface again a number of difficult issues in policy making for all blood transfusion services, including the difficulty of balancing a precautionary stance against other potential risk and opportunity costs, a lack of clarity on who is supposed to take the initiative leading often to a failure to take issues in the round and delays in policy making, and issues of the clarity of communication with the public, blood donors and blood recipients.

References:

1. Will RG, Ironside JW, Zeidler M et al. A new variant of Creutzfeldt-Jakob disease in the UK. Lancet 1996;347:921-25.
2. Zeidler M, Stewart GE, Barraclough CR et al. New variant Creutzfeldt-Jakob disease: neurologic features and diagnostic tests. Lancet 1997;350: 903-07.
3. Zeidler M, Johnstone EC, Bamber RWK et al. New variant Creutzfeldt-Jakob disease: psychiatric features. Lancet 1997;350:908-10.
4. Collinge J. Variant Creutzfeldt-Jakob disease. Lancet 1999;354:317-23.
5. Bruce M. New variant Creutzfeldt-Jakob disease and bovine spongiform encephalopathy. Nat Med. 2000;3:258-59.
6. Brown P, Will RG, Barclay R et al. Bovine spongiform encephalopathy and variant Creutzfeldt-Jakob disease: background, evolution and current concerns. Emerg Infect Dis 2001;7:6-16.
7. Lasmezas CL, Deslys JP, Demalmay R et al. BSE transmission to macaques. Nature 1996;381:743-44.
8. Collinge J, Sidle KCL, Meads J et al. Molecular analysis of prion strain variation and etiology of 'new variant' CJD. Nature 1996;383:685-90.
9. Bruce ME, Will RG, Ironside JW et al. Transmissions to mice indicate that 'new variant' CJD is caused by the BSE agent. Nature 1997;389: 498-501.
10. Hill AF, Desbruslais M, Joiner S et al. The same prion strain causes vCJD and BSE. Nature 1997;389:448-50.
11. Scott MR, Will RG, Ironside JW et al. Compelling transgenic evidence for transmission of bovine spongiform encephalopathy to humans. Proc Natl Acad Sci USA 1999;96:15137-42.
12. Cousens S, Vynnycky E, Zeidler M et al. Predicting the CJD epidemic in humans. Nature 1997;385:197-98.
13. Ghani AC, Ferguson NM, Donnelly CA et al. Predicted vCJD mortality in Great Britain. Nature 2000;406:583-84.
14. Ironside JW, Head MW, Bell JE et al. Laboratory diagnosis of variant Creutzfeldt-Jakob disease. Histopathology 2000;37:1-9.
15. Barclay GR, Hope J, Birkett CR et al. Distribution of cell associated prion protein in normal adult blood determined by flow cytometry. Brit J Haematol 1999;107:804-14.
16. Macgregor I, Hope J, Barnard G et al. The distribution of normal prion protein in human blood. Vox Sang 1999;77:88-96.
17. Hill AF, Butterworth RJ, Joiner S et al. Investigation of variant Creutzfeldt-Jakob disease and other human prion diseases with tonsil biopsy samples. Lancet 1999; 353:183-89.
18. Hilton DA, Fathers E, Edwards P et al. Prion immunoreactivity in appendix before clinical onset of variant Creutzfeldt-Jakob disease. Lancet 1998;352: 703-04.
19. Brown P. The pathogenesis of transmissible spongiform encephalopathy: routes to the brain and the erection of therapeutic barriers. Cell Mol Life Sci 2001;58:259-65.
20. Brown P, Cervenakova L, Diringer H. Blood infectivity and the prospects for a diagnostic screening test in Creutzfeldt-Jakob disease. J Lab Clin Med 2001;137:5-13.

21. Brown P, Rohwer RG, Dunstan BC et al. The distribution of infectivity in blood components and plasma derivatives in experimental models of transmissible spongiform encephalopathy. Transfusion 1998;38:810-16.
22. Brown P, Cervenakova L, McShane LM et al. Further studies of blood infectivity in an experimental model of transmissible spongiform encephalopathy, with an explanation of why blood components do not transmit Creutzfeldt-Jakob disease in humans. Transfusion 1999;39: 1169-78.
23. Rohwer RG. Titer distribution and transmissibility of blood-borne TSE infectivity. Cambridge Healthtech Institute 6th Annual Meeting. Blood Product Safety: TSE perception vs Reality. Virginia, USA. Feb 13-15, 2000.
24. Houston F, Foster JD, Chong A et al. Transmission of BSE by blood transfusion in sheep. Lancet 2000;356:999-1000.
25. Brown P. Transfusion medicine and spongiform encephalopathy. Transfusion 2001;41:433-36.
26. Andrews NJ, Farrington CP, Cousens SN et al. Incidence of variant Creutzfeldt-Jakob disease in the UK. Lancet 2000;356:481-82.
27. Cousens S, Smith PG, Ward H et al.: Geographical distribution of variant Creutzfeldt-Jakob disease in Great Britain, 1994-2000. Lancet 2001;357: 1002-07.
28. Bryant G, Monk P. Summary of the final report of the investigation into the North Leicestershire cluster of variant Creutzfeldt-Jakob disease. Leicestershire NHS Health Authority 2001.
29. Otto M, Wiltfang J, Schutz E *et al.* Diagnosis of Creutzfeldt-Jakob disease by measurement of S100 protein in serum: prospective case control study. B M J 1998; 316:577-82.
30. Miele G, Manson J, Clinton M. A novel erythroid-specific marker of transmissible spongiform encephalopathies. Nat Medicine 2001;7:361-64
31. Korth C, Stierli B, Streit P et al. Prion (PrPSc) specific epitope defined by a monoclonal antibody. Nature 1997; 390:74-77.
32. Fischer MB, Roeckl C, Parizek P et al. Binding of disease-associated prion protein to plasminogen. Nature 2000; 408:479-83.
33. Lee DC, Stenland CJ, Hartwell RC et al. Monitoring plasma processing steps with a sensitive Western Blot assay for the detection of the prion protein. J Virol Methods 2000;84:77-79.
34. Schmerr MJ, Jenny AL, Bulgin MS *et al.* Use of capillary electrophoresis and fluorescent labeled peptides to detect the abnormal prion protein in the blood of animals that are infected with a transmissible spongiform encephalopathy. J Chromatography 1999;853:207-14.
35. Safar J, Willie H, Itri V *et al.* Eight prion strains have PrP^{Sc} molecules with different conformations. Nat Med 1998;4:1157-65.
36. Roddie PH, Turner ML, Williamson LM. Leucocyte depletion of blood components. Blood Rev 2000;14:145-56.
37. Priola SA, Caughey B, Caughey WS. Novel therapeutic uses for porphyrins and phthalocyanines in the transmissible spongiform encephalopathies. Cur Opin Microbiol 1999;2:563-66.
38. Farquhar C, Dickinson A, Bruce M. Prophylactic potential of pentosan polysulphate in transmissible spongiform encephalopathies. Lancet 1999; 353: 117.

39. Korth C, May PC, Cohen FE et al. Acridine and phenothiazine derivatives as pharmacotherapeutics for prion disease. Proc Natl Acad Sci USA 2001; 98: 9836-41.

TICK-BORNE DISEASES: RECOGNIZED AND THEORECTICAL RISKS ASSOCIATED WITH BLOOD TRANSFUSION

David A. Leiby[1], Jennifer H. McQuiston[2] and Rodger Y. Dodd[1]

Introduction

Pathogenic microorganisms transmitted by ticks have taken on expanded public health significance during the last several decades. Ticks are now recognized to transmit over a dozen diseases that are caused by a variety of pathogenic agents ranging from bacteria and protozoa to viruses [1]. Humans have increasingly come in contact with ticks as they expand their outdoor recreational activities and move their homes to rural environments. Similarly, the reforestation of suburban neighborhoods has provided ideal habitats for transport and reservoir hosts (e.g., deer, rodents) of ticks and tick-borne diseases, further facilitating transmission to humans. During the same period, new etiologic agents of disease transmitted by ticks have emerged, while the geographic distribution of existing agents has expanded. Taken together, newly emergent tick-borne agents and those described previously pose an ongoing concern to public health.

While these agents are primarily transmitted to humans by ticks, the potential for several of these agents to be transmitted by blood transfusion has raised concerns for blood safety. The fact that many of these agents reside within blood cells and likely survive routine blood storage conditions suggests that they may be readily transmissible by blood transfusion. Indeed, several tick-borne pathogens have been reported to be transmitted by this route, and several others pose theoretical risks for transmission (Table 1). However, the extent to which these agents pose a threat to blood safety and what action, if any, is needed to prevent their transmission remains controversial. In large part, insufficient clinical and epidemiologic data are available to make informed decisions regarding the need for blood screening or other measures to protect the blood supply. Decisions are further hampered by the lack of licensed tests to screen blood for tick-borne pathogens.

In January 1999, a workshop entitled, "The potential for transfusion transmission of tick-borne agents", was convened in Atlanta, GA by the several U.S. government agencies (CDC, FDA, NIH, and DOD). The goal of this workshop was to provide those agencies entrusted with the safety of the blood supply

1. Transmissible Diseases Department, American Red Cross Jerome Holland Laboratory, Rockville, MD, USA.
2. National Center for Infectious Diseases, Centers for Disease Control and Prevention, Atlanta, GA, USA.

information and appropriate courses of action to reduce the risk of transfusion-transmitted tick-borne infections [2]. A summary of the workshop suggested that while information on many agents was limited, *Babesia microti* was clearly the agent of primary concern due to the significant number (>20) of reported transfusion-transmitted cases. However, in the ensuing three years, much has changed. The number of *Babesia*-related transfusion cases has more than doubled and now includes an autochthonous case from Japan and a second report of WA-1 transmission [3-5]. A presumptive transfusion case of human granulocytic ehrlichiosis (HGE), the first to date, has also been reported.(6) As for control measures, recent advances and in some cases implementation of leukoreduction and pathogen inactivation may now play a role in limiting potential transmission. Thus, in a relatively short period, issues pertaining to the transmission of tick-borne pathogens by blood transfusion have evolved dramatically.

Thus, while this paper will focus primarily on *B. microti*, other tick-borne agents known to be transmitted by blood transfusion and those theoretically transmissible will also be discussed. In addition, strategies for preventing the transmission of these agents, including risk factor questions, blood screening, leukocyte reduction, and pathogen inactivation will be explored.

Table 1. Tick-borne agents posing real or theoretical risks of transfusion transmission

Agent	**Disease**	**Cellular location**	**Transfusion cases**
Babesia microti	babesiosis	red cells	multiple
Ehrlichia chaffeensis	human monocytic ehrlichiosis	monocytes	none reported
Ehrlichia phagocytophila	human granulocytic ehrlichiosis	granulocytes	single case
Rickettsia rickettsii	Rocky Mountain spotted fever	endothelial cells	single case
Coltivirus	Colorado tick fever	red cells	single case
Flavivirus	tick-borne encephalitis	CNS	two cases
Borrelia burgdorferi	Lyme disease	plasma	none

The Babesia

The agents of human babesiosis, *Babesia* spp., are intracellular pathogens of red blood cells found throughout the world including the U.S., Mexico, Africa and Southeast Asia. Despite its apparent worldwide distribution, human cases are reported almost exclusively from Europe and the U.S. Since its first reported occurrence in 1966 [7], hundreds of cases of human babesiosis in the U.S. have been attributed to the rodent babesial parasite, *B. microti*. More recently, cases associated with *Babesia*-like organisms (e.g., MO-1, WA-1) have been reported in Missouri and the Pacific Northwest [8,9]. In Europe, human babesiosis is caused primarily by *B. divergens*, a cattle parasite, but human cases attributable to *B. bigemina*, *B. bovis*, *B. canis* and *B. microti* also have been reported [10].

Babesiosis is a zoonotic disease transmitted to humans primarily by ticks of the genus *Ixodes*. The primary vector for *B. microti* in the United States is *I.*

scapularis. The enzootic life cycles of *B. microti* includes the reservoir host, *Peromyscus leucopus*, commonly known as the white-footed mouse. Babesial infections generally are mild or subclinical, characterized by fever, headache, and myalgias that resolve within several weeks. More severe cases can occur in the immunocompromised patient (e.g., asplenic, elderly) and may be accompanied by hemolytic anemia, thrombocytopenia, renal failure and fatality rates of up to 5% [11]. Most cases of babesiosis are effectively treated with using therapeutic combinations such as quinine and clindamycin or atovaquone and azithromycin.

For most tick-borne pathogens there have been no or very few reported cases of transfusion-transmitted infection. In contrast, over 40 cases of *B. microti* transmission by blood transfusion have been reported during the last 20 years. In addition, two cases of transmission have also been attributed to the closely related WA-1 parasite, first reported less than 10 years ago [12]. Despite the worldwide distribution of *Babesia* spp., all reported transfusion cases have occurred in the U.S. with the exception of an autochthonous case recently reported in Japan [4]. Taken together, infected recipients have ranged in age from neonates to 79 years old and many were immunocompromised, including several who were asplenic. The incubation period in recipients was 2-8 weeks and diagnosis was usually made by identification of infected erythrocytes on blood smears, serologic measurement of antibodies to *B. microti*, or by PCR.

Table 2. Seroprevalence estimates for *Babesia microti* in selected populations

	n	%
Block Island, RI	574	9.0
Cape Cod*	779	3.7
Connecticut:	1,007	0.6
– *Borrelia* reactive	735	9.5
– Random	304	2.6
– College students	206	1.0
– No tick/Lyme exposure	40	2.5
Connecticut*	1,007	0.6
Long Island, NY	671	1.0
Shelter Island, NY	102	6.9
Shelter Island, NY	115	4.3
Wisconsin*	999	0.3

* Blood donor population.

In most transfusion cases red cell units have been implicated; however, at least four cases were attributed to platelet units which were likely contaminated with *Babesia*-infected red cells [2].

Seroprevalence estimates for *Babesia* spp. have been limited to the U.S. and range from 0.6% to 6.9% in some highly endemic regions of the Northeast, but few studies have included blood donor populations (Table 2) [2]. Those studies of blood donors suggest that 3.7% of Cape Cod, 4.3% of Shelter Island (NY), and 0.3-0.6 % of Connecticut donors had antibodies to *B. microti* [13,14, Leiby DA unpublished observations]. More recently, we conducted studies comparing the *B. microti* seroprevalence rate between 1,745 blood donors from *Babesia*-endemic and non-endemic areas of Connecticut. A significantly greater ($P < 0.002$) percentage of donors from the endemic area (1.4%) had antibodies to *B. microti* compared to donors from non-endemic areas (0.3%). Selected seropositive donors were evaluated for evidence of active parasitemia by PCR. Of the 19 seropositive donors tested, 10 (53%) were positive by PCR indicating the presence of active, ongoing infections with *B. microti* [Leiby DA unpublished observations]. This suggests that the potential risk of transfusion-transmitted babesiosis may be greater than earlier thought.

Other Agents

Several other tick-borne agents have been or are potentially transmissible by blood transfusion. Foremost among these agents are several rickettsial organisms; *Ehrlichia chaffeensis*, *E. phagocytophila*, and *Rickettsia rickettsii*. *E. chaffeensis* is the etiologic agent of human monocytic ehrlichiosis (HME), while *E. phagocytophila* causes HGE. As the disease names suggest, these agents have predilections for either monocytes or granulocytes, thus making them ideal candidates for transmission by transfusion. Based on empirical data, these two agents survive under blood bank conditions for between 11 and 18 days (Table 3) [15,16] Despite their intracellular location and survival in blood, no transfusion-transmitted cases have been reported for *E. chaffeensis*, while as mentioned previously, one presumptive case has been identified for the agent of HGE [6].

Table 3. Survival of tick-borne agents in blood

Agent (disease)	Transfusion case	Empirical study
Babesia microti (babesiosis)	35 days	21 days
Ehrlichia chaffeensis (HME)	NR*	11 days
Ehrlichia phagocytophila (HGE)	30 days	18 days
Rickettsia rickettsii (RMSF)	9 days	NR
Coltivirus (CTF)	8 days	14 days**
Borrelia burgdorferi (Lyme)	NR	48 days

* NR = none reported.

** Recovered from tubing attached to unit implicated in transfusion case.

This case occurred in Minnesota and involved a patient transfused with two red cell units. HGE infection was confirmed in the recipient by serology (titer of 1:512) and PCR. The implicated donor reported extensive deer-tick bites approximately 2 months prior to donation, and was found to be serologically positive for HGE at 1:2048. The implicated unit of red cells was transfused 30 days post-donation, thus the agent of HGE can survive in blood for up to 30 days, a much longer period than predicted by aforementioned empirical studies (Table

3). The recipient was treated with doxycycline and the symptoms resolved rapidly.

A single transfusion-transmitted case of *R. rickettsii*, the agent of Rocky Mountain spotted fever (RMSF), was prospectively identified in Baltimore following the diagnosis of RMSF in a donor three days post-donation; the donor died six days later [17]. A whole unit of this donor's blood, stored for 9 days at 4°C, was transfused to a patient who developed a headache and fever approximately 6 days post-transfusion. RMSF was subsequently confirmed in the patient by serology, animal inoculation and cell culture; the recipient was treated and fully recovered.

There have been three reported cases of tick-borne viruses transmitted by blood transfusion; one case involving the Colorado tick fever (CTF) virus and two involving the tick-borne encephalitis (TBE) virus, specifically Kumlinge. Like the RMSF case described above, the CTF transmission case implicated an infected Montana resident who had donated during the disease's incubation period.(18) The donor reportedly removed a tick 18 hours before donation, but did not develop an acute onset of fever until 3 days post-transfusion. Six days later testing confirmed that the donor had CTF. The transfusion service was notified of the donor's infection and tubing segments retained from the implicated donation (maintained at 4°C for 14 days) demonstrated CTF virus in the serum. A week earlier, blood from the infected donor had been transfused to an 82-year-old patient undergoing laparotomy. Following surgery the recipient experienced a prolonged febrile illness. CTF virus was detected in a cellular fraction of the recipient's blood 23 days post-transfusion. The infection subsequently resolved and the patient was released from the hospital. The details of the two cases involving TBE virus are sketchy at best, but both occurred on Kumlinge Island, Finland and involved a single donation [19]. As with the RMSF and CTF cases, the donor became ill shortly after donating blood and the recipients became febrile shortly after being transfused. The recipients were treated for symptoms with non-steroidal anti-inflammatory drugs and recovered rapidly.

Conspicuously absent from this discussion is *Borrelia burgdorferi* which has caused innumerable cases of Lyme disease in the U.S., Europe, and elsewhere. However, despite widespread reporting of infection and disease, to our knowledge no transfusion cases involving *B. burgdorferi* have been reported. On several occasions, donors have been diagnosed with Lyme disease shortly after donating blood, but unlike the RMSF, CTF, and TBE cases described above, evidence of infection was not demonstrable in the recipients [20]. This is in direct contrast to reports that experimentally inoculated *B. burgdorferi* spirochetes can survive in processed, banked blood through 48 days *in vitro* [21]. However, demonstration of spirochetes in patients with active Lyme disease has been difficult [22], suggesting that the spirochetemic phase may be very short. Thus, these and other as yet undescribed factors may play critical roles in preventing transfusion-transmitted Lyme disease.

Management Strategies

The limited number of epidemiologic studies and useful diagnostic/screening tests hinders the development of effective strategies to prevent the transmission of tick-borne pathogens. However, for some agents discussed herein, the absence or limited number of transfusion cases may suggest that no action is required at this time. For other agents, particularly *B. microti*, the large number of transfusion cases would seem to suggest that appropriate, agent specific strategies for preventing transmission are needed. Potential management strategies include risk factor questioning, blood screening, and product manipulation.

Existing blood safety strategies depend in part upon identifying at-risk donors by questions. In the case of tick-borne diseases, the fundamental risk factor for acquiring infection is contact with a tick vector. Thus, one approach to control transmission would be to defer all donors that report recent tick exposure. A regional survey of self-reported tick bites in U.S. blood donors indicated that many were capable of recalling recent bites [Leiby DA unpublished observations]. However, the frequency of tick bites in some regions approached 10%, a rate that would make deferral based on this question alone untenable. Alternatively, one could test donors reporting recent tick exposure, thereby targeting those at greatest risk, while greatly reducing the number of donors deferred. This approach was used in Connecticut to compare the seroprovelance of *B. microti* and *E. phagocytophila* in blood donors reporting tick bites versus control donors. For both agents, there was not a significant difference in seroprevalence rates when tick-bite and control groups were compared [Leiby DA unpublished observations]. However, since many persons infected with a tick-borne disease do not recall an associated tick-bite, the lack of difference should perhaps not be surprising. Moreover, individuals who report tick bites may be more vigilant in searching for and removing ticks. Because ticks generally need to feed 48-72 h to successfully transmit some infections, rapid removal of ticks may prevent transmission [23]. Thus, for these reasons, those donors reporting tick bites may actually be less likely to be infected than those who do not recall a tick bite.

The implementation of blood screening for any tick-borne pathogen remains problematic due to the lack of licensed blood screening tests. If tests become available, one of several strategies could be considered for implementation. As already discussed, one could use a risk factor question, but this approach does not appear to be viable. A second approach would be based on the present regional distribution of specific pathogens (e.g., *B. microti*). In this case, testing for a specific pathogen would occur only in those regions where the pathogen is endemic. While this approach may be more cost effective, it does not prevent a donor from being infected in an endemic area and then donating in a non-endemic area. For this reason, universal blood screening may be easier logistically. A final alternative would be to provide at-risk recipients blood products that have tested negative for tick-borne agents. A similar approach is presently used in the U.S. for management of cytolomegalovirus. As stated previously, most tick-borne agents cause relatively mild, self-limiting infections, but they can cause severe disease in at-risk recipients (i.e., elderly, immunocompromised). Thus, these at-risk recipients would be candidates to receive blood that has been tested and found negative for tick-borne agents.

The last approach to be considered is product manipulation, specifically pathogen inactivation and leukocyte reduction. The latter technique uses specialized filters to eliminate or decrease the number of leukocytes, which may in turn eliminate certain intracellular tick-borne agents. In particular, this technique may hold some promise in reducing rickettsial agents (e.g., *Ehrlichia*, RMSF) and feasibility has been demonstrated using the rickettsial agent of scrub typhus, *Orientia tsutsugamushi* [24]. This approach, however, would not be practical for intraerythrocytic pathogens such as *Babesia* and CTF virus. In contrast, pathogen inactivation via psoralens or other photosensitizing agents would theoretically be able to reduce or eliminate most pathogens regardless of their cellular location. These techniques have been validated using bacteria and viruses, but there have been few studies involving tick-borne agents and they have not been without complications. Indeed, a study targeting *B. divergens* reduced the overall parasite burden, but resulted in 0.1-0.5% lysis of red cells [25]. Although limited studies have been done to date, leukoreduction and pathogen inactivation offer alternative approaches to risk-factor questions or testing algorithms that need to be explored further.

Summary

During the past 20 years, tick-borne diseases have become an increasingly important threat to blood safety. New tick-borne diseases continue to be described, and the endemic ranges of known agents continue to expand. With increased recognition of these agents the number of transfusion cases has increased, particularly for *B. microti* and related *Babesia*-like parasites. Despite this increase in transfusion cases, educational and surveillance resources continue to lag for these and other tick-borne agents. Thus, an enhanced effort at securing epidemiologic data on these agents is needed. Similarly, the virtual absence of diagnostic and screening tests severely limits acquisition of new data and implementation of testing to ensure blood safety. While testing in some form may one day be implemented, the potential role of leukocyte reduction and pathogen inactivation also needs to be considered.

References

1. Spach DH, Liles WC, Campbell GL, Quick RE, Anderson DE, Fritsche TR. Tick-borne diseases in the United States. N Engl J Med 1993;329:936-47.
2. McQuiston JH, Childs JE, Chamberland ME, et al. Transmission of tick-borne agents of disease by blood transfusion: a review of known and potential risks in the United States. Transfusion 2000;40:274-84.
3. Cable RG, Trouern-Trend J. Tickborne infections. In: Linden JV, Bianco C, eds. Blood Safety and Surveillance. New York: Marcel Dekker, 2001:399-422.
4. Saito-Ito A, Tsuji M, Wei Q, et al. Transfusion-acquired, autochthonous human babesiosis in Japan: isolation of *Babesia microti*-like parasites with hu-RBC-SCID mice. J Clin Microbiol 2000;38:4511-16.

5. Fritz C, Hui L, Kjemtrup A, Thompson M. Tick-borne disease surveillance. In: 2000 Annual Report, Vector-Borne Disease Section, California Department of Health Services:20-22.
6. Eastlund T, Persing D, Mathiesen D, et al. Human granulocytic ehrlichiosis after red cell transfusion. Transfusion 1999;39(Suppl):117S.
7. Scholtens RG, Braff EH, Healy GR, Gleason N. A case of babesiosis in man in the United States. Am J Trop Med Hyg 1968;17:810-13.
8. Quick RE, Herwaldt BL, Thomford JW, et al. Babesiosis in Washington State: A new species of *Babesia*? Ann Intern Med 1993;119:284-90.
9. Herwaldt BL, Persing DH, Précigout EA, et al. A fatal case of babesiosis in Missouri: Identification of another piroplasm that infects humans. Ann Intern Med 1996;124:643-50.
10. Kjemtrup AM, Conrad PA. Human babesiosis: an emerging tick-borne disease. Int J Parasitol. 2000;30:1323-37.
11. White DJ, Talarico J, Chang H, et al. Human babesiosis in New York state. Review of 139 hospitalized cases and analysis of prognostic factors. Arch Intern Med 1998;158:2149-54.
12. Quick RE, Herwaldt BL, Thomford JW, et al. Babesiosis in Washington State: A new species of *Babesia*? Ann Intern Med 1993;119:284-90.
13. Popovsky MA, Lindberg LE, Syrek AL, Page PL. Prevalence of *Babesia* antibody in a selected blood donor population. Transfusion 1988;28:59-61.
14. Linden JV, Wong SJ, Chu FK, Schmidt GB, Bianco C. Transfusion-associated transmission of babesiosis in New York State. Transfusion 2000; 40:285-89.
15. McKechnie DB, Slater KS, Childs JE, et al. Survival of *Ehrlichia chaffeensis* in refrigerated, ADSOL-treated RBCs. Transfusion 2000;40: 1041-47.
16. Kalantarpour F, Chowdhury I, Wormser GP, et al: Survival of the human granulocytic ehrlichiosis agent under refrigeration conditions. J Clin Micro biol 2000;38: 2398-99.
17. Wells GM, Woodward TE, Fiset P, Hornick RB. Rocky Mountain spotted fever caused by blood transfusion. JAMA 1978;239:2763-65.
18. Randall WH, Simmons J, Casper EA, Philip RN. Transmission of Colorado tick fever virus by blood transfusion – Montana. MMWR 1975;24:422,427.
19. Wahlberg P, Saikku P, Brummer-Korvenkontio M. Tick-borne viral encephalitis in Finland. The clinical features of Kumlinge disease during 1959-1987. J Int Med 1989;225:173-77.
20. Cable R, Krause P, Badon S, Silver H, Ryan R. Acute blood donor co-infection with *Babesia microti* (Bm) and *Borrelia burgdorferi* (Bb). Transfusion 1993;33(Suppl.): 50S.
21. Johnson SE, Swaminathan B, Moore P, Broome CV, Parvin M. *Borrelia burgdorferi*: survival in experimentally infected human blood processed for transfusion. J Infect Dis 1990;162:557-59.
22. Shrestha M, Grodzicki RL, Steere AC. Diagnosing early Lyme disease. Am J Med 1985;78:235-40.
23. Mather TN, Telford SR, Moore SI, Spielman A. *Borrelia burgdorferi* and *Babesia microti*: efficiency of transmission from reservoirs to vector ticks (*Ixodes dammini*). Exp Parasitol 1990;70:55-61.

24. Mettille FC, Salata KF, Belanger KJ, Casleton BG, Kelly DJ. Reducing the risk of transfusion-transmitted rickettsial disease by WBC filtration, using *Orientia tsutsugamushi* in a model system. Transfusion 2000;40:290-96.
25. Grellier P, Santus R, Louray E., et al. Photosensitized inactivation of *Plasmodium falciparum*- and *Babesia divergens*-infected erythrocytes in whole blood by lipophilic pheophorbide derivatives. Vox Sang 1997;72:211-20.

XENO-TRANSPLANTATION AND XENOZOONOSES

E. Joost Ruitenberg[1,2,3]

Introduction

Transplantation of organs such as hearts or kidneys from one individual to another has become a highly successful mode of therapy. According to reports of the FDA (US Food and Drug Administration) and CBER (Center for Biologics Evaluation and Research) in the US ten patients die every day in the US, because a needed organ is not available to them. The supply of organs in the US is based on about 5.000 donors annually. The demands, however, rose from about 20.000 in 1990 to more than 60.000 patients waiting for organs in 1998. These huge needs stimulated research on xenografts as donor organs.

Xenografts fall into two categories, concordant, e.g. between non-human primates and humans, or discordant, e.g. from pigs to man. The consequences for transplantation are different. Discordant xeno-transplantation in an untreated recipient results in rejection of the organ in one to two hours. This is called hyperacute rejection or HAR. Concordant xeno-transplantation generally does not lead to HAR but to delayed xenograft rejection (DXR).

Xeno-transplantation leads to other concerns as well. They include the physiologic function compatibility of xenografts and the risk of xenozoonoses, i.e. infections caused by organisms transmitted from the animal donor organ to the human recipient [1].

In this short review first the history of xeno-transplantation including experiments with chimpanzee and baboon organs will be described, followed by a discussion on the risks of xenozoonoses in baboons. Next, results obtained with pig organs will be discussed followed by an analysis of xenozoonoses from pigs. After a section on the risks of xenozoonoses in general, finally some remarks on the future of xeno-transplantation will be made [based on reference 2].

History of xeno-transplantation

The use of concordant xenografts started with kidneys from chimpanzees and baboons. The Table provides an historic overview of the results [3].

---

1. CLB-Sanquin, Amsterdam, NL.
2. Department Biology and Society, Free University, Amsterdam, NL.
3. Department of Immunology, Fac. Veterinary Medicine, University of Utrecht, NL.

Conclusions which can be drawn from these data are the following:

In general these results are disappointing. Furthermore, it has become obvious that chimpanzees are not acceptable as organ donors for emotional and ethical reasons. Baboons are preferable, however there are a number of concerns - First, incompatibility of physiological functions between baboon and human organs. Next, baboon organs are too small for human adults. Although, some physiological functions of transplanted baboon organs will remain intact, others may not (e.g. insufficient levels of serum cholesterol). Finally, a major concern are the xenozoonoses.

Table 1. Use of concordant xenografts from chimpanzees and baboons

Donor	Organ	Outcome	Number of cases	Year
Chimp	Kidney	9 months	12	1964
Baboon	Kidney	10 days	1	1964
Baboon	Kidney	4.5 days	1	1964
Baboon	Kidney	2 months	6	1964
Chimp	Heart	1 day	1	1964
Chimp	Liver	14 days	3	1969-1974
Baboon	Heart	1 day	1	1997
Chimp	Heart	4 days	1	1997
Baboon	Heart	4 weeks	1	1985
Baboon	Liver	70 and 26 days	2	1983

Xenozoonoses in baboons

In general, there are three classes of highly risky organisms, i.e. bacteria, parasites and viruses, especially retroviruses. A strategy for avoiding these risks could be the screening and breeding of potential animal donors in specific pathogen-free (SPF) environments to avoid the risk of most bacteria, parasites and viruses. It is , however, almost impossible to avoid transmission of retroviruses, especially endogenous retroviruses existing already in the germ line with multiple copies.

Which are the problems related to retroviruses in the baboon genome? First, cross-species infection by retroviruses is considered possible. Next, simian immunodeficiency virus (SIV), similar to HIV-2, is probably non-pathogenic, but the virus can infect human peripheral blood lymphocytes in vitro. Furthermore, many exogenous retroviruses are able to infect baboons. One semi-endogenous retrovirus is BaEV belonging to C-type retroviruses. A recently identified cellular receptor for virus entry is also present on the surface of human cells, giving BaEV the potential to infect human cells during baboon-to-human xenotransplantation. Recently novel endogenous retroviruses have been identified, e.g. Papio cynocephalus endogenous retrovirus-PcEV [4].

These observations brought the FDA in 1999 to the following statement. Based on the fact that more than 20 known potentially lethal viruses, including Ebola virus, Marburg virus, Hepatitis A and B virus, Herpes viruses and retroviruses can be transmitted from non-human primates to humans the FDA concluded that the use of non-human primate xenografts raises substantial public health safety concerns:

- the public at large would be exposed to significant infectious disease risk;
- clinical protocols proposing the use of non-human primate xenografts should not be submitted to the FDA.

This ruling made the pig the only potential donor for xeno-transplantation.
Pigs and xeno-transplantation

There are various interesting aspects related to the use of pig organs for transplantation.

First, pigs are available in large numbers. Next, pigs share some elements of anatomy and physiology with humans. Pigs can be housed in SPF environments. They breed rapidly, allowing genetic manipulation, possibly making them more suitable donors. In the past several transplantations using pig cells, tissues and organs have been performed. They include foetal pig-to-human islet transplants for diabetic patients and foetal pig-to-human neural cells transplants for patients with Parkinson's or Huntington's disease. However, also with pig organs problems have been observed related to physiological and immunological incompatibility.

In the introduction the hyperacute rejection (HAR) was mentioned. Molecular mechanisms of HAR include binding of a large portion of pre-formed human natural antibodies and human complement and its regulatory proteins. Techniques have been developed to overcome HAR. They include the reduction of the levels of pre-formed antibodies in recipients, the development of transgenic pigs expressing human complement regulatory proteins. and recently the breeding of knock-out pigs lacking the 1,3 alfa-galactosyl gene responsible for a carbohydrate on pig cell membranes to which the human immune system strongly reacts.

Pigs and xenozoonoses

In pigs the most important pathogens are endogenous retroviruses which can not be screened out by traditional breeding methods or modern gene knock-out technology.

A porcine endogenous retrovirus (PoEV) has been identified in the domestic pig genome which is closely related to gibbon leukaemia virus and capable of infecting cells from various hosts in vitro, including cells from a human kidney cell line [5]. This virus was named PERV-PK and was capable of infecting human peripheral blood mononuclear cells [6]. Furthermore, multiple copies of PERV-A, -B, and -C have been observed in the pig genome [7].

The concern that PERV's could be cross-species transmitted from pig to human when using pig organs as xenografts have thus far been based upon results of in vitro experiments. However, recently the first evidence for ongoing PERV expression after pig pancreatic islet xeno-transplantation in vivo (in mice) has been obtained [8]. Thus, the concern for PERV xenozoonoses in immunosuppressed human patients should be taken seriously. Further concerns include the potential reactivation of endogenous retrovirus already existing in the host genome by recombination with exogenous virus. This is a potential concern because many retroviral sequences are present in the human genome (the human

ERV family). In this context the recent isolation of a novel porcine endogenous retrovirus (PERV-E) shown to be related to HERV 4-1) is highly relevant [9].

Risks from xeno-transplantation

From the aspects mentioned above it becomes clear that xeno-transplantation is not without risk. In various publications [1,2,10] concerns have been expressed. They can be summarised as follows [1]:

- Immunosuppression in xenografts recipients may enhance activation of latent pathogens;
- Organisms carried by xenografts may not be pathogenic in the native host species, but may cause disease in human recipients;
- Novel animal-derived organisms may cause novel and thus not recognised clinical syndromes;
- In the absence of diagnostic tools some organisms derived from non-human species may laed to increased public health risk.

Conclusions

Is there a future for xeno-transplantation in the light of ongoing novel developments in the area of biotechnology? In principle it should be possible to generate safe, well-tolerated and physiologically well-functioning xenotransplants. However, at this point in time this is not the case.

What should be the research agenda? First, it is clear that at this moment only pig organs have the potential to be used as xenotransplants. From the examples cited above the first challenge is to seek to generate PERV-free pig herds. In order to establish these herds more dedicated pig genome manipulation studies are needed. These studies should be accompanied by ongoing research into risks of cross species infection.

Next, appropriate cloning studies should be aimed at obtaining pig organs with no risk of rejection by the human recipient. An interesting example is the recent production of pigs lacking the 1,3 alfa-galactosyl gene.

And above all ongoing benefit-risk analysis is essential to establish public policies in potential risks and ethics of xeno-transplantation.

In the meantime the US-FDA plans establishing a register to archive xenograft patient and source-animal tissue samples and some countries, including the United Kingdom and the Netherlands have put xeno-transplantation on hold pending further research into risk of cross-species infection.

References

1. Michaels MG, Simmons RL. Xenotransplant-associated zoonoses.Strategies for prevention. Transplantation 1994;57:1-7.
2. Mang R. Endogenous retroviruses and xenotransplantation. PhD thesis, University of Amsterdam 2001 (pp. 127).
3. Steele DJ, Auchincloss HJ. Xenotransplantation. Ann Rev Med. 1995;46: 345-60.
4. Mang R, Goudsmit J, Van der Kuyl AC. Novel endogenous type C retrovirus in baboons: complete sequence, providing evidence for baboon endogenous virus gag-pol ancestry. J Virol 1999;73:7021-26.

5. Patience C, Takeuchi Y, Weiss RA. Infection of human cells by an endogenous retrovirus of pigs. Nat Med. 1997;3:282-86.
6. Wilson CA, Wong S, Muller J, Davidson CE, Rose TM, Burd P. Type C retrovirus released from porcine primary peripheral blood mononuclear cells infects human cells. J Virol. 1998;72:3082-87.
7. Le Tissier P, Stoye JP, Takeuchi Y, Patience C, Weiss RA. Two sets of human-tropic pig retrovirus. Nature 1997;389:681-82
8. Van der Laan LJW, Lockey C,Griffeth BC, et al. Infection by porcine endogenous retrovirusafter islet transplantation. Nature 2000;407:90-94.
9. Mang R, Maas J, Chen X, Goudsmit J,Van der Kuyl AC. Novel endogenous Type C retrovirus in pigs related to HERV-E: evidence for multiplication by inbreeding similar to PERV. Chapter V in reference 2.
10. Platt JL. Xenotransplantation: new risks, new gains. Nature 2000;407:27-30.

DISCUSSION

Moderators: S.L. Stramer and C.P.L. van der Poel

H.J.C. de Wit (Amsterdam, NL): Dr. Turner, you gave an overview of the developments of tests for Creuzfeldt Jacob disease – pre-clinical or clinical. That was very interesting, but I was not aware of the publication of the Israeli group who described a urine test this summer which looked very promising. I would be curious to know whether you know something more about this test. Could you tell us when we could expect a usable test in blood transfusion? Perhaps to be able to contain the sometimes draconian donor selection measures that we take now.

Secondly, if it is going to take some time to have a workable test available for blood screening, would it be feasible to invest more in tests that directly identify the prion, or in tests that might give a signal of pre-clinical stage of disease in donors. So, surrogate testing.

M.L. Turner (Edinburgh, UK): You are right, I did not mention the urine test mentioned. A lot of these assays actually look quite promising, the capillary electrophoresis looks promising, the Delfia approach looks promising, the Western blot is not bad and I think the urine test looks quite promising as well. The big problem is going to be trying to establish the specificity, sensitivity and validation in man, because as you know at anyone time we only have a relative small number of people who are alive with the disease, so getting hold of sufficient numbers of samples is not easy. When patients are they often have a very advanced dementia, so there are ethical issues about getting sufficient samples from them as well as practical issues. The difficulties in validating assays are particularly serious when you need to use infectivity studies which take quite a long time to complete. When will we have a test? I do not know the answer to that. There are some authorities such as Paul Brown who think that a peripheral blood assay is not going to be possible because of the sensitivity issues I described to you. There are others who are a lot more optimistic, some have commercial optimism to back them and others do not. I think assays are looking pretty promising and are starting to go in the right direction. Personally I think In the next few years we will see a preliminary assay come along, but then our problem is going to be in deciding that we have got a sufficient specific assay to implement. What are we going to tell people if we do not really know much about specificity and sensitivity. When we get the preliminary assay than we are really going to get difficulties.

The final part of your question is yes – I think a surrogate assay is therefore well worth exploring. The EDRF story is extremely interesting. It seems possible that is telling us that there are subtle pathological changes in the haematopoietic system which might be utilizable as a reflection that there is some kind of disease ongoing. Of course, what we need to know is an awful lot more about EDRF; what kind of conditions it can be disturbed in and what its normal ranges are in a general population. So, I think there are some possibilities out there, but I do not know when we can expect an implementable assay.

R.Y. Dodd (Rockville, MD, USA): Could I just follow up on that question. You also talked about potential impact on the donor population. I think there have been some estimates from the UK that in fact the availability of such a test might have an impact on people's willingness to donate.

M.L. Turner: Yes, I think this is a big worry. A preliminary evaluation of donors is being carried out asking them questions such as: If there was an assay would you be prepared to have it undertaken and would you like to know the results or not? I am sure we have been here before in many respects. The thought of as a blood donor being told "Well, you have an abnormal PrPc result; we do not actually know what that means, it could mean that you are going to develop a very nasty brain disease sometime in the future". What impact is that going to have on your life insurance and your mortgage and so on? I would imagine we would see a significant hit amongst donors who may not be prepared to come forward and take the test.

C.Th. Smit Sibinga (Groningen, NL): Could I follow this up. Dr. Dodd, yesterday in his opening presentation talked about the phenomenon that we have a number of agents but no disease which makes it difficult. Here we have a very peculiar situation: There is a disease and there is an agent, but we do not know whether there is a relation between the two in the human setting. So, we are going to test eventually for an agent and we try to link that to a disease. How would you look at that, because that is kind of an odd phenomenon now?

M.L. Turner: Yes, it is an odd phenomenon, I agree. There is definitively an association between PrPsc and infectivity. Whether PrPsc is itself the infective agent is still argued about by the experts in the best field. The predominant feeling is that there are pathophysiological links, but there are still a significant number of experts in the TSE field who think it is nucleic acid protected by the conformation of the molecule that is conveying the disease. Certainly the link between presence of PrPsc and infectivety is not necessarily one to one or stable. If you look at different strains of TSE and in different animals, the ratio between infectious units and PrPsc molecule is not fixed. You can get PrPsc which does not appear to be infectious. For example, PrPsc can be generated in vitro in cell free systems but has not been shown to be infectious. So, there is more to it I think than just a lump of PrPsc. There are other components which we do not yet fully understand. So, in a sense I guess PrPsc is to some extend a surrogate marker of infectivity itself.

C.Th. Smit Sibinga: Should we then look at the introduction of such a test more as an opportunity rather than a precaution?

M.L. Turner: We cannot do infectivity assays on everybody obviously and the time frames involved are not practical for screening purposes. PrPsc is probably the best we are going to have.

C.Th. Smit Sibinga: Dr. Kortbeek, you came to the conclusion, based on the science behind it, that toxoplasmosis is not really a risk in blood transfusions. Yet we ask our donors and we exclude our donors. Would you be prepared to find that a redundant question to be asked donors?

L.M. Kortbeek (Bilthoven, NL I do not know exactly what the procedure is for donors at the moment; you do screen donors?

C.Th. Smit Sibinga: No, we just ask the question

L.M. Kortbeek: What kind of question do you ask?

C.Th. Smit Sibinga: Well, if you have had toxoplasmosis in the past.

L.M. Kortbeek: So and how do they know?

C.Th. Smit Sibinga: Some do, most do not.

L.M. Kortbeek: No, because it is hard to know only those patients who have a congenital infection will know. That is a very small proportion. I do not think there is a good question to ask. Risk factors are eating raw meat, especially from animals coming from outside their own barn and have lot of fecal contact with cats. Those people are more likely to be positive for toxoplasmosis. You have to do a serological test and in the Netherlands there is no regulation for testing pregnant women. We have no screening program for that. Some European countries do have that. In France for example you have to do it before you can get married. However, many women are not married before they get pregnant. In Austria screening for toxoplasmosis during pregnancy is obligatory by law; the test assigned is an immunofluorescence test. Nobody knows why that test has been picked out. But it does not prevent people getting infections. So, I do not think there is any rationale for screening. If you want to screen you have to consider what you want to know. Asking questions is no use, because we do not know the real risk factor yet. In the Netherlands we performed a risk factor study. We know there is a regional difference if you live in the Noord Holland – so in the neighborhood of Amsterdam – you have about a 3 fold higher risk than living in the South, but that is only for elderly people. Young people originating from that area are not at a greater risk. So, there is something in the region we do not understand, but there is something. It could be what is on the menu. Although we are a small country, there is a lot of difference in the food items we eat. It could be that, but we do not know and we cannot ask that to people..The only thing we can do is testing.

C.Th. Smit Sibinga: So, actually a redundant question therefore?

L.M. Kortbeek: Yes, I think so..

C.Th. Smit Sibinga: Prof. Ruitenberg, an extremely interesting presentation. I think it hit the nail on the head. Specifically against the background of what recently has been decided in the Netherlands regarding xeno-transplantations. There was another aspect which I thought you were going to talk about – the revival of xeno-immunoglobulines, for instance equine immunoglobulins. How about that?

E.J. Ruitenberg (Amsterdam, NL): That is a very good question. There are still a lot of countries in the world using horse or equine immunoglobulins either for prophylactic or for therapeutic reasons. We talk about for instance anti-tetanus, anti-rabies, anti-snake venom immunoglobulins. There is !! clearly a need in these countries. I am talking about Southeast Asia but also parts of Africa where there is not enough human immunoglobulin, particularly specific immunoglobulin available. Discussions have been held under the auspices of the World Health Organization and it is anticipated that for the coming 10 to 15 years horses will be in high demand to produce these antisera. In order to make sure that horse viruses or parasites are not transmitted to man, there are some programs in the countries for instance in Thailand where they still use horse immunoglobulins. They screen for infectious equine anemia, caused by a virus, which has not been proven to !!be a zoonosis. There are also parasites for instance Treponema equiperdum, which is present in Thailand and in Vietnam. What they do is look for evidence of the viruses or parasites and that is still for the next 10 to 15 years to continue in my opinion.

C.L. van der Poel (Amsterdam, NL): Yesterday we discussed already the scientific background of donor questionnaires. To my recollection actually in the new guidelines toxoplasmosis is not in the questionnaire. So, and that is good, but there is another thing which is still in the questionnaire.

Dr. Marcelis, we still ask donors whether they have had dental treatment. The assumption is that you would get a bacteriemia. Is that realistic, because you once told me that there might be other occasions where you develop bacteriemia as well and that might not be very significant as compared to dental treatment. Could we take the question off the questionnaire or is it reasonable to keep it in?

J. H. Marcelis (Tilburg, NL): Well, it is all based on the basic phenomenon that bacteria can cross not intact barriers. I told you once that everybody who just cleans up his teeth develops for a short time bacteriemia – about half a minute or something like that. But if you have a very intense dental procedure the gums are of course defected and that will stay for much longer time. That is the reason why it is good to wait until the gums are healed again. But there are of course many other situations where we do not ask for and where the risks of transportation of bacteria are much higher for instance the complete gastrointestinal tract. The mouth is just the beginning of the gastrointestinal tract and most bacteria are found in the colon. In clinical situations you see positive blood cultures of patients having for instance gastrointestinal carcinoma in which the defective mucous membrane of the gut is the place of the small locus where the bacteria come in the blood stream. In any such gastrointestinal information it would be safer not to use the blood donated.

H.T.M. Cuypers (Amsterdam, NL): Dr. Marcelis, regarding the special bags you are using to sample the first volume of blood. You were showing that is was only a reduction of 70% of the number of bacteria. Does it make sense to spend money manufacturing this more expensive bag and have only a reduction of 70%? Because we should probably think in reduction of logs when thinking about bacterial safety measures.

J.H. Marcelis I think it is more complicated than that; it is not only a reduction but as you could read from the information from Cecile Bruneau[1], it is also a change in the composition of the bacteria which were left. I think that Henk Olthuis[2] has already proven that many years before that following disinfection especially the bacteria on the surface of the skin are wiped out and the bacteria in the deeper layers of the skin are still left. Our results are in accordance with his findings. So, it can be seen that the most pathogenic bacteria are not originating from the normal flora, but originate from the transient flora. If you are only able to partly disinfect the skin and then separately collect and throw away the first punctured core of the skin, I think you do something good. What is left are bacteria from the deeper inner layers of the skin and those are diphteroids and other species which will result in lesser problems.

S.L. Stramer (Gaithersburg, USA): I like to continue the discussion about bacteria and talk about bacterial detection. Obviously, to do testing and not to distribute is the most effective method of eliminating any bacterially contaminated blood product. You indicated that, in the Netherlands you do culture immediately after collection and incubate 48 hours prior to distribution of product, but then you continue to culture I believe it is for 7 days, although I do not know if you went in to that. Than you do a recall if necessary. My question is the logic behind that. When you distribute the product my assumption is the product would be used in the hospital. So, what you are 'recalling' is basically a notification of the recipient that they received a bacterially contaminated product. The question or the discussion that I would like to pose is the logic of doing that. Why not as you distribute the product terminate your bacterial culture at 48 hours. Whatever you prevent, which I assume it would be the majority, would grow out in 48 hours. So, I would like to pick your brain about that.

---

1. Bruneau C, Perez P, Chassaigne M, et al. Efficacy of a new collection procedure for preventing bacterial contamination. Transfusion 2001;41:74-81.
2. Olthuis H, Puylaert C. Methods for removal of contaminating bacteria during venapuncture. ISBT Venice 1995; poster abstract 13.

J.H. Marcelis: I think that is because we had two objectives to start culturing. First, to prevent bacterial contamination and transfusion-submitted infections. But it is also a part of our hemovigilance program. I am eager to know whether there are other bacteria of which we do not know at this moment that they are present in high numbers, can grow after five days and could be transfused. But I agree that there will be some fuss if you call to the hospital after seven days and say: 'Well, how is your patient, we find a possibly complete innocent bacterium after seven days of culture'. But maybe, because we do not know, the physician will say: 'Well that is very interesting because there is a patient with an in line catheter and it is colonized'. When you find back the same bacteria then I say bingo. Maybe after a few years we will stop culturing at the moment the transfusion has taken place. That should be rational, but that is when we know what is happening. That is my point of view.

C.Th. Smit Sibinga: Actually the logic is in the monitoring for an issuing criterion; it is not a criterion for release from quarantine but an issuing criterion. The moment you find a unit positive in this culture technique – a carbon dioxide release color change technology – that unit is taken out of the stock and discarded. The units that remain on the shelf are still eligible for issuing. So, the moment you have a request you could then look at your stock, check with the monitor whether everything is still ok and then release. That is what Dr. Marcelis also showed in his presentation. It has a cost effectiveness aspect and it really weighs out the costs for the testing. We are doing this in Groningen since about four years. Mr. de Wit and I started that as a criterion and had to convince the hospitals that the extra charge for all this testing would pay off because there would be much more excess to platelet issuing than before.

S.L. Stramer: But my question is the logic of continued culture. I understand the issue of hemovigilance.

C.Th. Smit Sibinga: No, you do not continue on the same unit; that flask is taken out, but you continue on the units that are still on the shelf.

This is how we have done it so far, because if the unit has been found positive that was of no further issuing use.

C.L. van der Poel: I think this is a very interesting issue because actually during the Vienna ISBT meeting we had a meeting of the infectious diseases working party. Well, this was exactly the subject: How do you handle the logistics, how do you go on culturing for seven days. To my perception there are two extra arguments for continuing culturing for seven days – it is a large amount of blood products that is been cultured then and the seven days might also pick up slow growing bacteria that might be present in the red cells. In the medical advisory board in the Netherlands there were discussions about whether not to inform the treating physicians of the fact that they have received possibly infectious red cells, that already have been transfused. The discussion was more or less dominated by the clinicians who said: 'Well, I would want to know even if it is only just a screening test and we have to wait for the confirmation some days later in the identification'. If you have a patient and there is fever and if you then know that there might be infectious red cells, there are things you can do'. For bacteria there are treatment regimes. So, it is a totally different picture from viral notification like hepatitis C or hepatitis B. It were exactly the clinicians who were in favour of being notified. So, I think we will have to move on with these logistics and find out in close relation with our clients and our hospitals and discuss with them as we go on with this new guidelines. How can we handle it, is this a good way to do it or are there better ways. Dr. Marcelis, do you have to add anything on this issue?

J.H. Marcelis: No, we discussed it many times and yes that is all.

C.L. van der Poel: But there are big differences; as the report comes out from the working party[1] one may notice that there is a large difference about the opinions. There is one opinion though which was a bit interesting: If pathogen inactivation comes can we then abandon bacterial screening. That is one question and the other question was since the parasitologists already moved to PCR why not also the bacteriologists?

J.H. Marcelis: Maybe we should do that too, but I do not know how it is with parasites. Are you sure that bacteria which you detect in blood in PCR are still alive? I think that is maybe an important question. Maybe someone who does many PCR's does know more about that. I do not know whether when you look at parasites you restrict yourself to toxoplasma and to malaria for instance. However, when I want to look to bacteria there are about a 200 million types of bacteria. I do not know whether just RNA PCR is the solution for this.

C.L. van der Poel: But maybe then dedicated PCR's for some 8 or 10 agents that we find most often in these cultures?

J.H. Marcelis: Maybe in the next ten years when we got those nice biochips, which all the potent pathogens are already mapped in.

C.L. van der Poel: So, it is not wanted dead or alive with the bacteria then.

L.M. Kortbeek: I think it is one of the advantages of looking at bacteria that you have a test like 16S RNA, because we do not have that in parasites. Parasitic diseases are more complicated with regard to that. So, I think you are lucky if you want to look at that. If that is positive you can go on discovering what it is – active or not or still alive. So, all we have is our specific DNA-test and not the overall test like 16S RNA. I think you can use that as a screening and if it is possible you go on and you can use messenger RNA and things like that. So, look at whether they are active or not.

1. ISBT Working Party on Transmissible Diseases, Vienna 2000.

J.H. Marcelis: On bacteria we are also looking to ribosomal nucleic acid which is in many copies present in the material, so you do not need a multiplication step. Maybe that is promising for the next future.

C.L. van der Poel: So, that will be very handy then in terms of releasing. Dr. Dodd, I know you have presented some ideas about pathogen inactivation versus bacterial screening. Is there any caveat hat we have to look into when we enter that discussion in the coming two years. Where do we have to be really looking at before we make a decision to abandon bacterial screening when we introduce only pathogen inactivation for platelets and we culture only the platelets. Could you then stop culturing the platelets or are there some issues we have to look at.

R.Y. Dodd: The data that I have seen suggest that existing pathogen inactivation methods would be expected to do a very good job on bacteria because they are only going to be present at a few logs at the stage when you would do the inactivation process. So, I think it is reasonable to look at that as an alternative to culturing. Culturing is in a difficult kind of situation, because at some places as Dr. Marcelis showed, the requirement is really just a quality control requirement and in others it is being turned into a screening requirement with quality control aspects built in. I happen to think that it is a difficult situation, a difficult thing to implement in a full GMP environment, because basically you are deliberately throwing away some of your information in doing a screening test of that type. What you are trying to do is a sterility test and most formal sterility tests now take 14 days. So, it becomes very difficult to figure out exactly what you are doing. You are doing a partial solution and that is fine. But in our environment if we try to explain to the FDA why we had released a platelet product that we subsequently found by our own procedures to be contaminated with bacteria, I think it would be a difficult discussion.

H.T.M. Cuypers: I do not completely understand this information to the hospitals. You are now culturing in platelet pools, so when you have one positive there are 5 or 6 six red cell erythrocyte products to be traced. Are you then informing all these five hospitals or the recipients of these red cell products, because probably only one is infected?

J.H. Marcelis: You are right, but as we expect that the cultures of the platelets will be at a very early time positive or stay negative, it is the question whether all the individual red cells are already issued and transfused to patients. I am not sure about that. At least our blood bank always tries to issue the oldest red cells to the hospitals and that is a good Dutch system. So, in many cases I think not all the red cells are already out of the blood bank and when they come into the hospital the same Dutch practice is done again by the head of the transfusion laboratory. They give again the oldest red cells to the patients. So, I think in many cases we will trace the red cells in the blood bank or we will trace it at the transfusion center in the hospital itself. Seldom we may have to say to the doctor 'Sorry, your patient got a product which could be infected with a 20% chance'.

Even that is not a real problem, because in erythrocyte concentrates the same bacteria are isolated but on a much lower frequency than from platelets from the same donation.

III. TRANSMISSIBLE DISEASES

NAT UPDATE; WHERE ARE WE TODAY?

Susan L. Stramer[1]

Update of yield

A recent review covered the one-year experience with NAT in North America [1]. In that review, five different programs including testing with two different manufacturers of NAT assays for both HIV-1 and HCV were discussed. When combined, the HCV yield for 16.3 million donations tested was 62 confirmed positives (1:263,000); the HIV-1 yield for 12.6 million donations tested was 6 (1:2,100,000). Two of the six HIV-1 NAT positives were also HIV-1 p24 antigen (Ag) reactive; excluding those donors that were already detected by an FDA licensed screening test for p24 Ag reduced yield to 1:3,150,000. Updating these numbers for two years of screening increases the number of yield samples for HCV to 113 per 29,253,815 donations screened (1:259,000) and for HIV-1, including HIV-1 p24 Ag reactives, to 8 per 26,339,192 donations screened (1:3,292,400). Excluding the two HIV-1 p24 Ag reactives reduces the HIV-1 NAT yield to 6 (1:4,390,000). The updated numbers for the two-year experience are shown in Tables 1 and 2. Variability observed by site for HCV NAT yield is influenced greatly by the HCV antibody-screening test used. For sites using HCV 2.0, their yield is approximately 1:150,000 whereas sites using HCV 3.0 have yields that range from 1:300,000 to 1:500,000 (March 2001, FDA Blood Products Advisory Committee, BPAC, Meeting).

In addition to monitoring for yield performed under INDs, tracking also occurs for the number of false-positive donations and consequently that of deferred blood donors. As discussed at the March 2001 BPAC meeting, there are two sources of NAT false positivity; at the pool level or at the individual donation level. The 0.18% rate of false-positive pools observed for the American Red Cross' (ARC) NAT program is defined as those pools whose reactivity cannot be reproduced from testing the constituent donations; the undiluted sample represents the "gold standard". The rate of unresolved pools is comparable to the initial reactive rate in serologic testing. The rate of false-positive donations, corresponding to the loss of the donor, since donor reinstatement algorithms have not been approved by the FDA, is approximately 1:25,000 for the ARC

1. Executive Scientific Officer, National Testing and Reference Laboratories and Blood Services American Red Cross. 9315 Gaither Road, Gaithersburg, MD 20877. stramers@usa.redcross.org.

Table 1. NAT yield - Approximate two years of screening (March/April 1999-June 2001)

SITE (Program)	No. donations tested	NAT-positive, seronegative HIV-1	HCV
ARC (TMA pools 128→16)	14,003,704	4 (1*)	53
ABC (TMA pools 24→16)	5,136,858	3 (1*)	23
AIBC (TMA pools 24→16)	776,173	0	4
ABC	8,144,660	NA	32
(Roche pools 16)	6,422,457	1	NA
CBS (Roche pools 16)	1,192,420	NA	1

* Two p24 Ag confirmed positive.

Table 2. NAT yield - Approximate two years of screening (March/April 1999-June 2001)

No. donations tested	NAT-positive, seronegative HIV-1	HCV
29,253,815	NA	113 (1:259,000)
26,339,192	8* (1:3,292,400) 6 (1:4,390,000)	

* Two p24 Ag confirmed positive.

Table 3. Summary of NAT at the ARC

Parameter (No.)	128-member pools 3/3/99-9/7/99	16-member pools 9/8/99-5/29/01
Screened	2,338,304	11,665,400
Pools tested	18,268	727,983
Unresolved pools (%)	25 (0.14%)	1,341 (018%)
HCV yield	7 (1:334,043)	46 (1:253,600)
HIV Yield	0	*4 (1:3,500,000) Total study
Sum of all false positive seronegative donations	0	479 (1:24,400)

* One p24 Ag confirmed positive.

Table 4. NAT false-positive donor yield - Approximate first year of screening (March/April 1999-June 2000)

SITE (program)	No. donations tested	No. deferred donors
ARC (TMA pools 128→16)	7,700,000	187 (1:28,650)
ABC (TMA pools 24)	2,340,000	486 (1:4,800)
AIBC (TMA pools 24)	375,000	93 (1:4,000)
ABC (Roche pools 24)	4,800,000 1,600,000	195 (1:24,600) HCV 4 (1:400,000) HIV
Total	15,215,000	965 (1:15,800)

NAT program (Table 3). Rates of false positivity vary by program and by site and the overall number reported for the US was 1:15,800 for the first year of testing ([1]; Table 4).

True versus false NAT reactivity is determined by several strategies. Firstly, most programs will retest a NAT-reactive donation either by the same NAT method or a "supplemental" NAT method. Supplemental NAT is defined as a NAT method of a different technology or at minimum uses the same technology but with different primers and probes. In addition, most programs attempt to obtain an independent sample from the donation; i.e., either another sample tube or the plasma unit. In either case, NAT and serology are repeated to confirm the original test-of-record results.

One study performed by ARC to determine if NAT reactive unresolved pools represent false positivity looked at the signal strength of pools that did not resolve versus those that did resolve from 9/8/99 to 2/25/01 (Figure 1). For 3,023 pools that resolved to a single NAT-reactive donation, the mean signal to cutoff (S/CO) ratio was 9.84 (95% confidence interval of 9.74 to 9.94) whereas the mean S/CO ratio for those 1,212 pools that did not resolve was 3.73 (95% confidence interval of 3.55 to 3.91). In order to answer the question regarding the significance of those pools that did not resolve to a single reactive donation, the donors associated with the 1,212 pools were followed regarding their sero-status and NAT status for any subsequent donations (N=19,392; Figure 2). For 17,232 donations that could be tracked as from ARC donors, 7,666 made subsequent donations (over a median interval of 87 days; range 3 to 457 days). All donations tested NAT negative and none confirmed positive for any infectious disease marker. However, three donations did test as repeat reactive in either HIV-1 p24 Ag or HIV-1/HIV-2 antibody testing but all were serologic false positives. In addition 28 donations again were contained in NAT-reactive, unresolved pools. All 28 donations tested NAT non-reactive when tested individually. Of the 28 donors testing reactive twice in unresolved pools, eight had made a third donation. All eight tested negative by serologic testing and NAT in pools on the third donation. In conclusion, no true reactivity could be associated from NAT-reactive pools that did not resolve to individual donation.

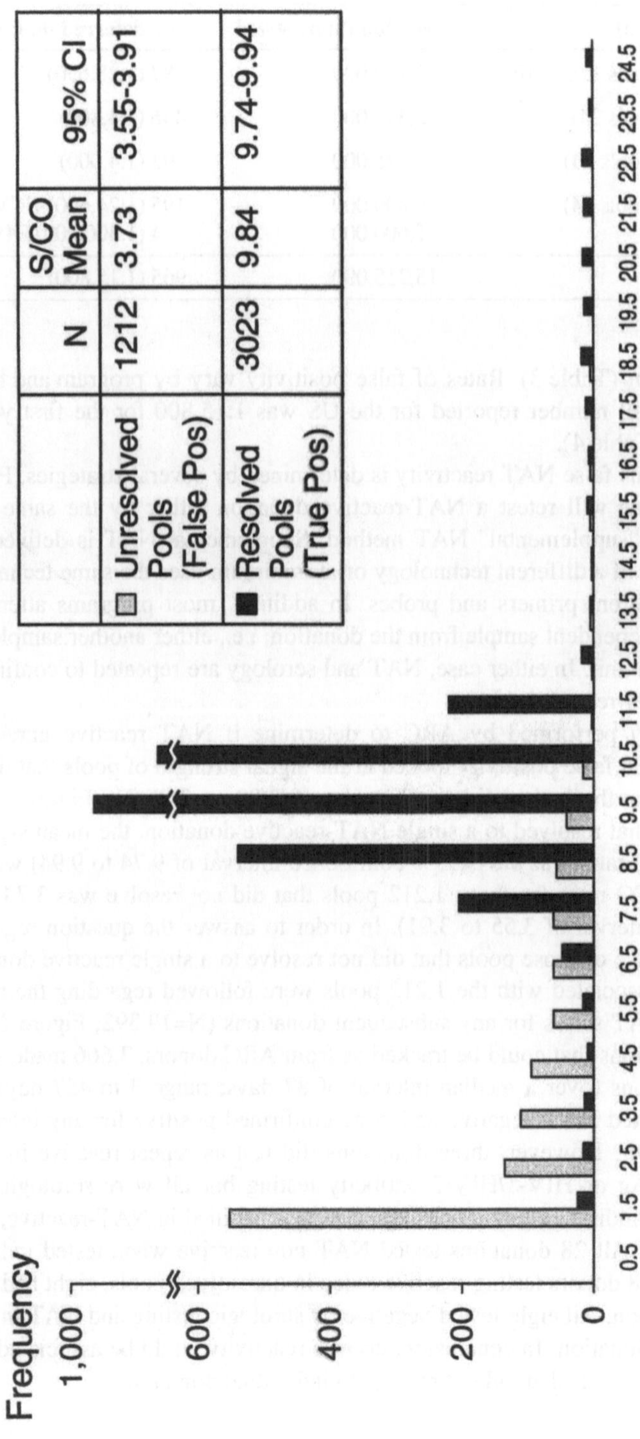

Figure 1. NAT-reactive pool resolution testing – ARC (9/8/99-2/25/01).

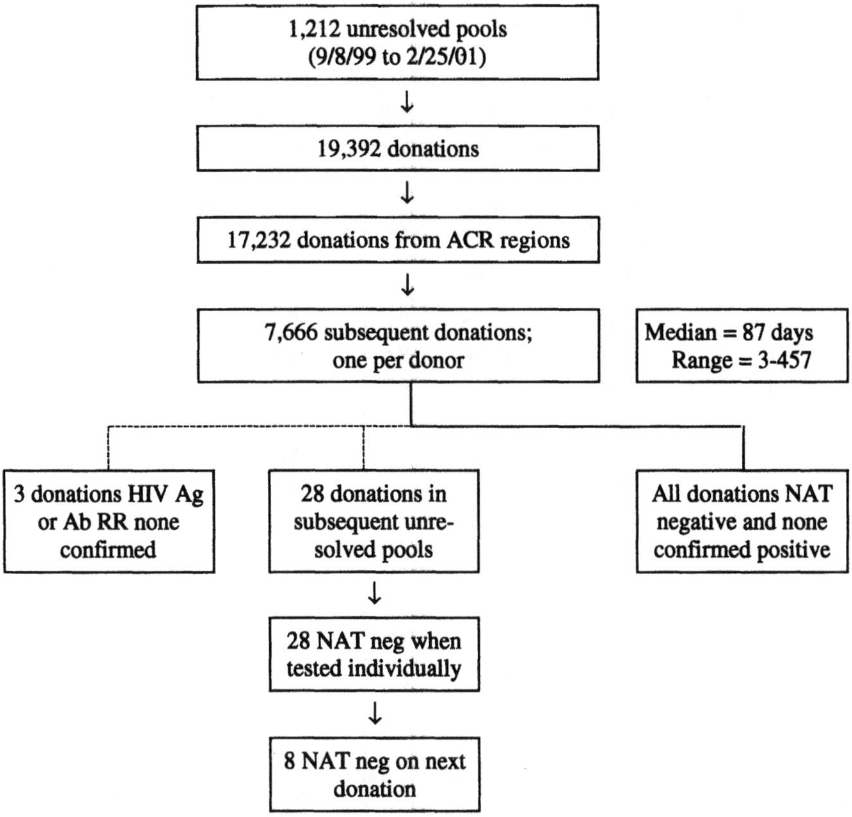

Figure 2. NAT-unresolved pools do not contain samples from HIV or HCV infected individuals.

Details of HIV yield samples

For three HIV NAT confirmed-positive donors, follow-up samples were available through seroconversion (Table 5). Two of the three donors were identified only by NAT at index whereas, one of the three was identified by NAT and p24 Ag. The p24 Ag-positive, NAT-positive sample was the sixth HIV antibody-negative donor identified as p24 Ag reactive at index at the ARC since the implementation of p24 Ag screening in March 1996. At 6.5 million annual collections, six p24 antigen confirmed positive, seronegative donations is a yield for 5 years of just over 1 per year or 1 per 5.4 million. All samples collected from the three HIV NAT confirmed-positive sero-converting donors were RNA positive by TMA and PCR; the sample having the highest viral load was the peak antigenemic sample in all cases. Following the decline to negativity of p24 Ag, RNA still remained positive. Earlier detection and longer persistence of RNA indicate that RNA reactivity is a more sensitive marker of HIV infection than p24 Ag [2]. In each case of seroconversion, the first HIV western blot-positive sample lacked a band at p31 and contained bands to only p24 and gp120/160. Although representing true infection in these three cases, donors having HIV western blot positive results that lack a band at p31 are frequently

Table 5A. Comparison of HIV-1 NAT-positive window-case U.S. blood donors - ARC

SC	Sample collection (days)	RNA Copies/mL	p24 s/CO	Percent neut.	HIV-1/ HIV-2 Ab S/CO	WB
1	Index	**$2.1{\times}10^3$**	0.30		0.07	
	5	**$4.0{\times}10^5$**	**1.22**	111	0.12	
	11	**$6.0{\times}10^5$**	**4.19***	102	0.86	
	42	**$1.1{\times}10^5$**	0.81		**15.25**	POS minus p31
2 (6)	Index	**$7.5{\times}10^5$**	**5.35**	94	0.05	
	7	**$2.1{\times}10^6$**	**13.90**	96	**2.18**	IND
	14	**$4.7{\times}10^5$**	**2.56**	95	**2.76**	IND
	21	**$8.5{\times}10^4$**	0.82		**3.09**	IND
	31	**$3.9{\times}10^4$**	0.13		**8.66**	POS minus p31
	37	**$3.5{\times}10^4$**	0.18		**13.04**	POS – all bands
	45	**$4.6{\times}10^4$**	0.27		**14.61**	POS – all bands
3	Index	**390**	0.31		0.79	IND
	6	**350**	0.33		**1.81**	IND
	16	**$3.8{\times}10^4$**	**2.52***	90	**3.19**	POS minus p31
	24	**$1.3{\times}10^5$***	**13.55**	83	**5.78**	POS minus p31

false positive [3]; additional data discussing false-positive HIV western blots are discussed later.

Replacement of p24 antigen screening by NAT

The three HIV sero-converting donors identified in pools of 16 by NAT, of which only one was p24 Ag reactive at index, coupled with the duration of time that RNA was positive prior to, and during, seroconversion as compared to p24 Ag both indicate that p24 Ag testing could be replaced by NAT. Further studies have been performed to demonstrate that p24 Ag could be eliminated in lieu of NAT. Three seronegative samples identified by p24 Ag prior to NAT implementation at the ARC were diluted in negative defibrinated human plasma and tested by NAT at dilutions up to 1:128; all diluted samples were strongly NAT reactive (Table 6). Samples from HIV NAT yield cases detected in pools of 16 to 24 were similarly found NAT reactive at a dilution of 1:128. Samples identified at index that were both HIV NAT and p24 Ag positive had higher viral loads than those that were identified only by NAT; i.e., greater than 100,000 copies/mL if both RNA and p24 Ag positive versus 2,000 to 20,000 copies/mL if only RNA positive. These data also indicate that NAT is a more robust indicator of HIV infection than p24 Ag.

Another study focusing on a larger population compared the sensitivity of p24 Ag and NAT in HIV antibody, confirmed-positive samples. Of 580 allogeneic donations confirmed positive for HIV antibody from 9/8/99 to 2/28/01 from

Table 6. Detection of HIV-1 p24 Ag and NAT yield samples by HIV-1 NAT (1:128 dilutions)

Case	Index detected by	Index RNA conc. undiluted (copies/mL)	Multiplex 1:128* (S/CO)
ARC 2	Ag	6×10^5	+ (16.08)
ARC 3	Ag	1×10^5	+ (16.06)
ARC 5	Ag	3×10^5	+ (29.59)
Milwaukee (Ag-)	NAT	2×10^4	+ (7.86)
ARC 1 (Ag-)	NAT	2×10^3	+ (7.99)
ARC 6 (2)	Ag/NAT	7.5×10^5	+ (21.99)

* Diluted in RNA screened negative defibrinated plasma.

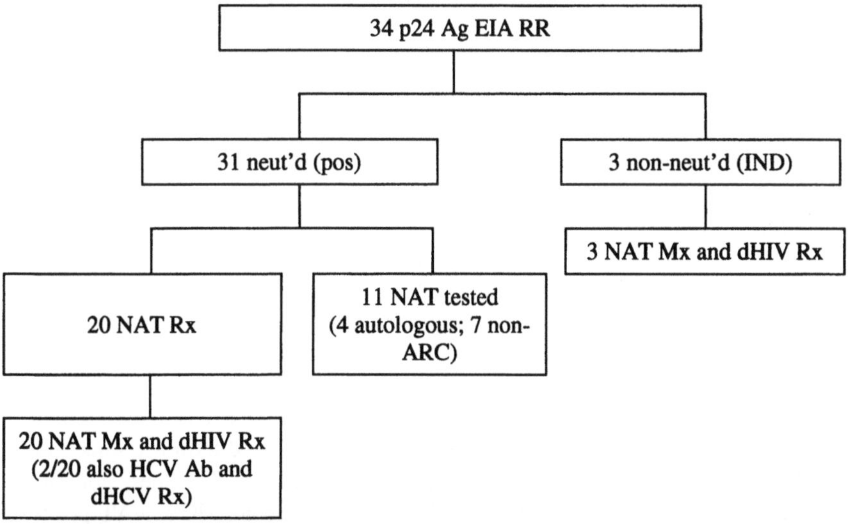

Figure 3. NAT/p24 Ag analysis of HIV-1 WB confirmed-positive samples (9/8/99 to 2/28/01) (N=580 NAT performed at ARC or allogeneic = 321).

testing performed at the ARC, 34 were p24 Ag repeat reactive with 31 confirmed positive by neutralization (Figure 3). Of those 31, 20 were NAT reactive by TMA in both the multiplex and discriminatory tests; the remaining 11 were not NAT tested either because the donations were autologous or not NAT tested by the ARC. Interestingly three of the p24 Ag indeterminate; i.e., non-neutralized, samples were also NAT reactive indicating that the neutralization test failed to detect three virus-containing samples. Of the 580 HIV antibody-positive donations, 321 could be compared directly for reactivity to NAT and p24 Ag since these donations were tested for all HIV markers by the ARC (Figure 4). Of the 321 HIV antibody-confirmed positive donations, 304 were NAT positive including the 20 that were confirmed positive for p24 Ag (Figure 3). Therefore, there were 284 HIV antibody-positive donations that were p24 Ag negative but detected by both HIV/HCV multiplex and HIV discriminatory NAT. There were no samples that were detected by p24 Ag that were not detected by NAT.

		p24 Ag		
		Pos	**IND or Neg**	**Total**
NAT Mx and dHIV	**Pos**	**20**	**281 (neg)** **3 (RR→ IND)**	**304**
	Neg	**0**	**17**	**17**
	Total	**20**	**301**	**321**

Figure 4. NAT/p24 Ag analysis of HIV-1 WB confirmed-posituve samples (9/8/99 to 2/28/01) (N=580 NAT perfomed at ARC or allogeneic = 321).

Details of HCV yield samples

During the ARC NAT screening program from 3/3/99 to 5/29/01, 53 HCV NAT reactive, seronegative donors have been identified (Table 7). Of those, 48 were confirmed by PCR at index, 33 were confirmed by testing an independent sample from the plasma unit and 27 were confirmed by a follow-up sample. Of those that enrolled in follow-up studies, 19 have sero-converted in a mean time of 42 days. Of the total 53, 29 (55%) were male, 27 (51%) were repeat donors; the mean age was 34 years (range 17-71). Seventeen (32%) had an ALT eleva tion above 120 IU/L with 15 continuing to have an elevated ALT value at sero-conversion. With HCV NAT in place, ALT screening of blood donors has no value for the detection of early HCV infection.

One genotype 2B, HCV-infected, seronegative donor has been immune-silent for 587 days (Table 8). The donor has been followed monthly since index NAT reactivity. The donor continues to have normal ALT values, consistent NAT reactivity by TMA and high viral loads [4]. Another HCV NAT-positive immune-silent donor, genotype 3A, has been sampled monthly for over 340 days without seroconversion. The second immune-silent donor also has consistently normal ALT values and high viral loads ranging from 220,000 to 5.5

Table 7. Characteristics of 53 HCV NAT confirmed-positive donors (5/29/01)

No. confirmed by			**Sex**	**Donor status**	**Mean age**	**No. ALT elevated at index**
PCR at index	Plasma	FU	29 M	27-Rpt	34	>60=25
48	33	27 (19 of 27 sc'ted at mean of 42 days)	24 F	26-FT	(17-71)	>120=17 +15 at SC

Table 8. Characteristics of an HCV NAT reactive immunosilent donor

No.	Site	Donor status	Sex	Age	Collection date	ALT	S/CO MP	PP	WBN	Disc	Supplemental NAT (Quant., Genotypes)
7	Columbus, OH*	Rpt	M	44	08/21	20	*8.43*	*9.73*	*9.38*	*22.05*	4,300,000 2B
	follow-up 7 (202 days)					24			*10.13*	*22.05*	8,600,000
	follow-up 8 (235 days)					22			*12.26*	*22.95*	11,000,000
	follow-up 9 (263 days)					17			*10.24*	*20.96*	3,600,000
	follow-up 10 (299 days)					19			*10.97*	*21.37*	4,800,000
	follow-up 11 (362 days)					22			*9.51*	*19.63*	2,900,000
	follow-up 12 (424 days)					14			*11.79*	*21.34*	7,700,000
	follow-up 13 (529 days)					13			*8.93*	*27.57*	1,400,00
	follow-up 14 (587 days)					22			*9.11*	*21.45*	11,000,000

* Donor had been incarcerated, exposed to blood from wife, friend IDU.

million copies per mL. Both donors test negative on both FDA licensed antibody screening tests for HCV.

Resolved HCV NAT reactivity has been observed in two donors; however, one of the two was NAT negative for 100 days prior to seroconversion. One HCV NAT reactive donor has what is believed to be an abortive infection. This 40-year old female donor was infected with genotype 1A/1B with a viral load of 8,400 copies per mL. Her viremia was twice confirmed in the index plasma unit but on four follow-up samples, collected up to 131 days after index, neither NAT reactivity by TMA or PCR nor seroconversion could be demonstrated. All samples from the index testing and follow-up samples were the same blood type and had identical HLA patterns eliminating the possibility of sample mix-up. The profiles for follow-up sampling (indicated by vertical lines) including seroconversion for all HCV NAT confirmed-positive donors is shown on Figure 5. Viral loads at index in the 53 NAT confirmed-positive donors identified to 5/29/01 at the ARC ranges from 100 to 51 million copies/mL, with a median viral load of 2.7 million (Table 9). Multiple genotypes have been identified for seronegative NAT positives with the greatest frequency, as expected in the US

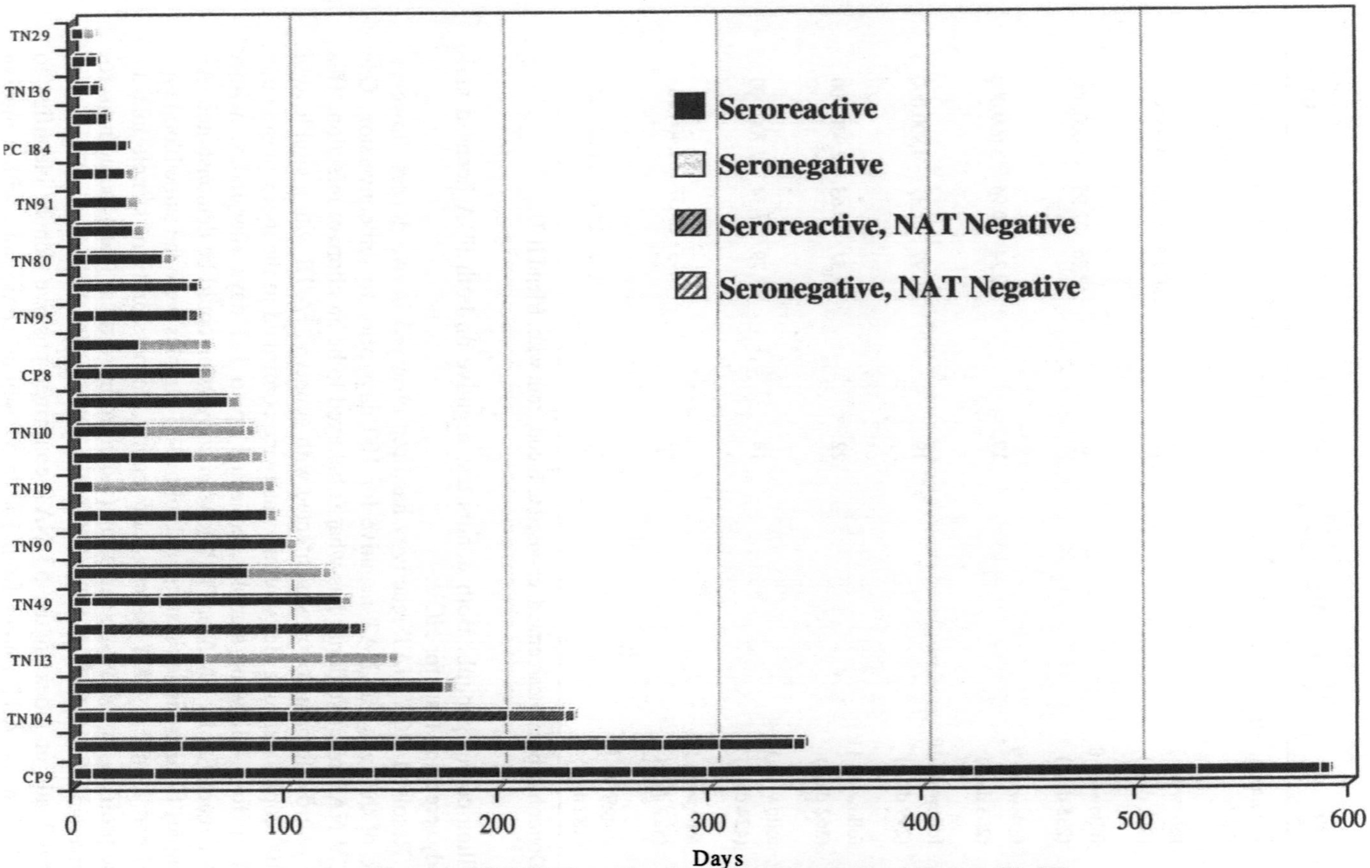

Figure 5. HCV NAT reactive donations confirmed by follow-up (N=27).

Table 9. Characteristics of 53 HCV NAT confirmed-positive donors compared to HCV serology confirmed-positive donations (5/29/01)

Viral load	Genotype distribution	
100-51,000,000 Median=2,700,000	1A, 1B = 31	
	2A = 1 2B = 10 3A, 3B = 9 6A = 1	42% non 1A, 1B genotypes
Seropos viral load 200-39,000,000 Median=2,650,000	1A, 1B = 132	
	2A = 4 2B = 25 3A = 10	23% non 1A, 1B genotypes

[5,6], occurring for genotypes 1A and 1B (58%). The viral loads and genotype distributions for 171 random donor samples selected over the same period of time that were HCV antibody confirmed positive (Ortho 3.0 repeat reactive and positive by RIBA 3.0) are similar to what has been observed for NAT. However, genotypes 1A and 1B appear to occur at a higher frequency (77%) in the sero-positive group; this observation may be the result of relative small numbers in the comparison.

Comparisons of NAT and serology results – relevance for donor counseling

Routine NAT screening data are useful for confirming the infectious disease status of HCV and HIV EIA repeat reactive donors, and should be incorporated into donor notification and counseling programs. Data for the first year of NAT screening, from 9/8/99 to 8/31/00, in which serology repeat reactive samples were included into pools for testing by NAT demonstrate correlation between serology confirmatory testing status and NAT.

For HCV, a total of 7,868 samples were repeat reactive of which 4,566 (58%) were confirmed by RIBA 3.0; of those, 80% were NAT positive (Table 10). This number is consistent with reports that approximately 15 to 20% of HCV-infected individuals will clear infection [7,8]. The NAT-negative samples that confirmed positive by RIBA could therefore either represent:

- resolved infection,
- false negativity by NAT, or
- RIBA false positivity.

Due to the close agreement between percentages, it seems likely that the vast majority of these samples represent resolved infection. Re-testing of the 913 NAT-negative, RIBA-positive samples was performed; 2% of samples screened in pools were reactive when tested individually by PCR but less than 1% of

Table 10. Correlation of NAT screening with supplemental HCV serological results (8,476 RR donations of which 7,868 (93) were available for RIBA) (9/8/99 to 8/31/00)

NAT result	RIBA result			Total
	Pos	Ind	Neg	
Pos	3,653 (80%)	62*	34** (2,5%)	3,749
Neg	913	1,153	2,053	4,119
Total	4,566 (58%)	1,215	2,087	7,868

* 43/62 (76%) dHCV and PCR Rx.
** 5/34 (15%) dHCV and PCR Rx.

Table 11. Correlation of NAT screening with supplemental HCV serological results (4,232 RR donations of which 4,043 (95.5%) were available for RIBA) (9/8/99 to 8/31/00)

NAT result	Western Blot result			Total
	Pos	Ind	Neg	
Pos	213 (94%)	38*	21** (1.5%)	272
Neg	913	1,901	1,856	3,770
Total	226 (5.6%)	1,939	1,877	4,042

* 2/38 (5%) dHCV and PCR Rx.
** 0/21 (0%) dHCV and PCR Rx.

those samples tested individually by TMA were PCR positive when re-tested [9]. Of the total NAT reactive samples following initial TMA screening, 2.5% were RIBA-indeterminate or RIBA-negative. Of those, 43 of 62 (76%) RIBA indeterminates and 5 of 34 (15%) of RIBA negatives confirmed as NAT reactive following discriminatory TMA and PCR. The total number of RIBA- indeterminate samples that could be confirmed as NAT reactive totaled 43 of 1,215 (3.5%), whereas the number of RIBA-negative samples totaled 5 of 2,087 (0.2%). Therefore, the overall agreement between confirmed HCV NAT positiv iity and RIBA positivity is very high (3,701/3,749=98.7%). If the requirement to perform RIBA testing were eliminated for NAT reactive samples, the consequence would be a small number of NAT reactive donors provided with a false-positive message.

For HIV, a total of 4,042 samples were repeat reactive of which 226 (5.6%) were confirmed by western blot; of those, 94% were NAT positive (Table 11). NAT reactive, western blot-indeterminate and negative samples following initial NAT screening included 38 indeterminates and 21 negatives, totalling 1.5% of the total NAT screen reactives. However, with the exception of two indeterminate

Table 12A. Characteristics of HIV-1 WB Pos/TMA neg samples (9/8/99 to 8/31/00)

Sample	Pool	Neat	HIV-1/HIV-2 S/CO	WB	HIV PCR
1		NR	1.43	41,120,160	Neg
2	Nr		1.03	41, 160	Neg
3		NR	1.62	41, 160	Neg
4		NR	.1.11	41, 55, 160	Neg
5		NR	12.50	24, 41, 51, 61, 160	Neg
6		**NR**	**20.18**	**all bands**	**Neg**
7		NR	1.22	24, 41, 160	Neg
8			1.11	17, 41, 120, 160	Neg
9	NR		1.84	41, 160	Neg
10	NR	NR	1.40	24, 41, 160	Neg
11		NR	1.70	17, 24, 41, 51, 160	Neg
12	**NR**		**20.00**	**all bands**	**Pos (200 copies/mL)**
13		**NR**	**17.84**	**all bands**	**Neg**

All samples –24 Ag negative.

Table 12B Characteristics of HIV-1 WB Pos/TMA neg samples (9/1/00 to 4/23/01)

Sample	Pool	Neat	HIV-1/HIV-2 S/CO	WB	HIV PCR
14		NR	8.73	17, 24, 160	Neg
15	NR		10.56	24, 51, 120, 160	Neg
16	**NR**		**19.30**	**all bands**	**Neg**
17	**NR**		**19.47**	**all bands**	**Pos (100 copies/mL)**
18			4.73	41, 160	Neg

All samples –24 Ag negative.

samples, none had NAT reactivity confirmed by discriminatory NAT or PCR testing. There were 13 western blot positive, but NAT non-reactive samples that could only be explained as either NAT false negative or western blot false positive. Table 12A provides a line listing for the 13 samples; Table 12B pro vides data for an additional five samples from 9/1/00 to 4/23/01 that were also western blot confirmed positive but NAT non-reactive. Most of these western blot positive samples, because of known serology reactivity at the time of pooling, were screened by NAT individually. Three samples listed in Table 12A have high screening results (S/CO values) and also have all bands present on western blot. In contrast, the remaining samples had low S/CO values of 2.50 or less and all lacked a p31 band on western blot. Approximately one half of samples lacking a band at p31 have been determined to represent false positivity on the western blot and all samples containing only bands to envelope have been determined to be false positive [10]. None of the ten antibody weakly reactive samples could be confirmed by PCR when an independent sample was tested individually and therefore are likely to be falsely western blot positive (Table 12A). Of the three strongly reactive, antibody-confirmed positives, one was PCR positive; however, the viral load was low (200 copies/mL). Similar results are provided for the additional five samples listed in Table 12B; one of two strongly antibody-confirmed positive samples was PCR positive with a very low viral load (100 copies/mL). Therefore, probable HIV true positive samples may have very low viral loads or be RNA negative on NAT screening assays.

Estimates of residual risk and cost

NAT yield for the first year of testing at the ARC was compared to the estimated yield using the model, yield is the product of incidence (per hundred thousand, pht) and the window period (wp) in days closed by NAT [11,12]. Estimates of HCV window-period reduction as a consequence of NAT detection prior to antibody reactivity has been calculated to be between 40 and 59 days of the total HCV antibody-negative window period of 70 days using HCV 3.0 antibody assays [13,14]. Using a calculated HCV incidence in repeat ARC donors from 1998-1999 [15] of 2.24 pht projects an annual NAT yield in repeat donors of 14.7 to 22.1 or 21.6 to 32.8 depending on the window periods used [16]. The actual yield for the first year of NAT screening at the ARC was 15 NAT confirmed-positive donors, which lies within the 95% confidence interval of the estimate using the window period of 40 days. Using the 15 NAT yield samples and derived incidence calculation, the window-period closure obtained by NAT was calculated at 32.5 days (range of 27 to 41 days). Both the 40 and 32.5-day calculation of window-period reduction agree with the two-year data for NAT confirmed-positive yield cases that have been followed through seroconversion; those data as shown on Table 7 were 19 of 27 donors seroconverted in a mean of 42 days. HCV incidence in first-time donors may be estimated using the calculated window-period reduction for NAT of 32.5 days and the actual NAT yield of 14 in first-time donors for one year. The calculation predicts an HCV first-time donor incidence of 7.45 pht as opposed to 2.24 pht in repeat donors. Previously there have been no reports of methods to estimate incidence for HCV in first-time donors. Although the estimated incidence in first-time donors is approximately 3-fold greater than in repeat donors, the NAT yield in first-time and repeat donors is similar due to the higher percentage of repeat donors.

Table 13. Annual estimates for HCV (+95% C.I.). Generated by NAT for first-time and repeat donors

Yield	Incidence	WP (days)
18.4 (± 3.7) - Rpt Est.	2.24 (± 0.46)	40
27.2 (± 5.6) - Rpt Est.	2.24 (± 0.46)	59
15 - Rpt yield	2.24 (± 0.46)	32.5 (27-41)
14* -FT yield	7.45 – Inc. Est.	32.5 WP Est.

* Among an estimated 2.11×10^6 first-time donors.

Table 14. Viral incidence and window period projections

	Incidence in repeat donors (pht)	WP-NAT	WP + MP NAT	WP + SD NAT
HIV	1.72	16	11	7
HCV	2.24	70	10	7
HBV	4.46	45	39	20

Table 15. Calculated risk per million RBCs transfused

	- NAT	+ MP NAT	+ SD NAT
HIV	0.75 (1:1,300,000)	0.52 (1:1,900,000)	0.33 (1:3,000,000)
HCV	4.3 (1:230,000)	0.61 (1:1,600,000)	0.43 (1:2,300,000)
HBV	5.5 (1:180,000)	4.8 (1:210,000)	2.4 (1:410,000)

Table 16. Calculated benefits by type of infection avoided

	QALY per infection avoided	Infections avoided per year (QALYs)	
		MP ←serology	SD ←serology
HIV	7.1	3.5 (25)	6.4 (45)
HCV	0.60	55 (33)	58 (35)
HBV	0.16	11 (1.7)	46 (7.2)
Total		(60)	(87)

Table 17. Calculated benefits by type of infection avoided

	Cost effectiveness ($ Million) QALY	Maximum cost ($)/donation for ≤$50,000/QALY	
MP NAT HIV/HCV	2.7	0.22	
MP NAT HIV/HCV/HBV	3.2	0.23	$102-192 million (cost of total QALY per infection avoided)
MP NAT HIV/HCV/HBV – p24 Ag/anti-HBc	1.7	7.23	
SD NAT HIV/HCV/HBV – p24 Ag/anti-HBc	1.6	7.34	$139 million

* Assumes $12.00/donation (MP) and $15.00/donation (SD) NAT for HIV/HCV and $3.00/donation for HBV NAT

The ARC calculations of HIV, HCV and HBV incidence and window-period reductions estimated 1) prior to NAT (WP-NAT), 2) post NAT using mini-pools of 16 to 24 donations (WP+MP NAT) and, 3) post NAT if single donation screening were employed (WP+SD NAT) are provided in Table 14 (17,18). For HIV, approximately one-half of the total viremic window period will be closed by pooled NAT versus the vast majority of window-period reduction for HCV. In contrast because of low viral loads and a slow doubling time for HBV early in infection, window-period reduction using mini-pool screening is small. A greater impact for window-period reduction would occur with individual donation screening using tests of high sensitivity. However, even with individual donation HBV NAT screening, there is still a calculated 20-day window period due to low viral load samples that may not be reliably detected by NAT. The status of mini-pool HBV NAT yield relative to current and improved methods of HBsAg screening were discussed at the March, 2001 FDA BPAC meeting. Data were presented demonstrating the low yield of HBV NAT relative to next generation HBsAg screening assays having 0.1 ng/mL or better sensitivity.

Using these numbers, residual risk for all three agents may be calculated (Table 15). Current risk post mini-pool NAT for HIV is estimated at 1:1,900,000; for HCV residual risk is reduced from prior to NAT at 1:230,000 to 1:1,600,000 post mini-pool NAT. HBV risk estimates range from 1:180,000 currently since HBV NAT is not performed to 1:210,000 for mini-pool NAT and 1:410,000 for single donation NAT [17]. The numbers for HBV residual risk and NAT yield will require additional validation in prospective studies in the US where both HBsAg and anti-HBc screening are performed. Precise estimates for HBV residual risk and consequently the benefit of NAT are difficult to calculate due to the transient nature of HBsAg reactivity and the non-specificity of the current anti-HBc assays.

The calculations of residual risk in Table 15 can be used to predict the benefit in terms of quality-adjusted life years (QALY). Table 16 shows the QALY estimates per infection avoided for each agent [17]. QALY varies by severity of disease that results following infection, the cost of treatment and possibility of cure, the chances of chronic carriage, etc. Therefore, calculations of QALY are highest for HIV, intermediate for HCV and lowest for HBV, where the least disease burden and cost to society exist. Using the QALY estimates and number of infections avoided by either mini-pool or individual donation NAT, the total QALY can be calculated for both NAT methods.

Table 17 compares four different screening strategies and the cost effectiveness of each expressed as cost per QALY in millions of US dollars. The four NAT strategies listed represent ranges of what may occur over time. They include mini-pool NAT for HIV and HCV with and without HBV. The cost effectiveness of mini-pool NAT ranges from $2.7 million per QALY without HBV to $3.2 million with HBV. The cost calculations assume $12.00 per donation for mini-pool screening and $15.00 per donation for individual donation screening for HIV/HCV with an additional $3.00 added per donation for HBV. HIV/HCV/HBV mini-pool NAT cost effectiveness was also evaluated with the theoretical elimination of two current serological tests: p24 Ag (already discussed) and anti-HBc, which may be redundant once HBV NAT is implemented. Eliminating these two current serological tests decreases the cost for mini-pool NAT for all three agents from $3.2 to 1.7 million per QALY [18]. If one were then to move to single donation NAT for all agents with the elimination of the redundant tests for HIV and HBV, the cost effectiveness would actually improve from $1.7 to 1.6 million because of the additional HIV infections detected. Discussions of QALY have used a cutoff of $50,000 to define the limit of cost effectiveness; i.e., if cost were above the $50,000 cutoff, the intervention was determined not to be cost effective. Using this cutoff, calculations of the maximum amount that NAT per donation should cost were determined. If redundant screening tests were no longer performed, the NAT cost per donation could be significantly higher, consistent with existing NAT pricing and still be cost effective. Overall calculations for the cost of mini-pool NAT per year in the US are $102 to 192 million depending on agents included and whether all current serological testing is retained. The cost of individual donation NAT for all agents with the elimination of p24 Ag and anti-HBc screening is estimated at $139 million.

Conclusions

Although not currently cost effective using traditional measures, NAT implementation has reduced the residual risk for both HIV and HCV in the US to numbers that are extremely low and approach one per two million donations screened. The impact of NAT on the number of lost donors and products has been small due to low false-positive rates and validated algorithms [19]. NAT yield and false-positive rates in the US and Canada have been consistent over time as well as relatively consistent between programs and even comparable to the European experience with NAT [20]. The most significant factor contributing the HCV NAT yield appears to be whether HCV 2.0 or 3.0 antibody screening assays are used. HCV seroconversion in NAT confirmed-positive donors is variable with a mean of 42 days; however, two donors followed for one year or longer have remained immune-silent. For HIV, although NAT yield is very small, seroconversion patterns are highly reproducible. These data, as well as data from many other studies comparing p24 Ag to HIV NAT, demonstrate that p24 Ag testing should be eliminated once HIV NAT is licensed by the FDA. NAT has also been demonstrated to be very useful when coupled with HIV and HCV serologic results since NAT serves to increase the positive predictive value of the final donor result. The outlook for HBV mini-pool testing is uncertain because of predicted low yields; for HBV NAT to be successful in terms of maximum yield, the assays will have to be highly sensitive and most likely will involve individual donation testing that will require automated systems with cGMP features.

Acknowledgements

Thanks are given to Sally Caglioti (Blood Systems Laboratories), D.M. Strong, PhD (Puget Sound Blood Center), Richard Gammon, MD (America's Independent Blood Centers) and Vito Scalia (Canadian Blood Service) for kindly sharing their NAT experience (Tables 1, 2 and 4).

References

1. Stramer SL, Caglioti S, Strong DM. NAT of the United States and Canadian blood supply. Transfusion 2000;40:1165-68.
2. Stramer SL, Porter RA, Brodsky JP, et al. Replacement of HIV-1 p24 antigen screening with HIV-1 RNA nucleic acid testing (NAT) for whole blood donations. Transfusion 1999;39:10S.
3. Kleinman S, Busch MP, Hall L, et al. False-positive HIV-1 test results in a low-risk screening setting of voluntary blood donation. JAMA 1998;280: 1080-85.
4. Peoples BG, Preston SB, Tzeng JL, et al. Prolonged antibody-negative HCV viremia in a US blood donor with apparent HCV transmission to a recipient. Transfusion 2000;40:1280-81.
5. Lau JYN, Mizokami M, Kolberg JA, et al. Application of six hepatitis C virus gentotyping systems to sera from chronic hepatitis C patients in the United States. J Infect Dis 1995;171:281-89.
6. Zein NN, Persing DH, Hepatitis C genotypes: Current trends and future implications. Mayo Clin Proc 1996;71:458-62.
7. Alter HJ, Seeff LB. Recovery, persistance, and sequelae in HCV infection: A perspective on long-term outcome. Semin Liver Dis 2001;20:17-35.
8. Seeff LB. Why is there such difficulty in defining the natural history of hepatitis C? Transfusion 2000;40:1161-64.
9. Stramer SL, Brodsky JP, Peoples BG, et al. Relationship of nucleic acid testing (NAT) results to HIV and HCV serology among donors; relevance to counseling. Transfusion 2000;40:115S.
10. Stramer SL, Kleinman SH, Busch MP. Rate of HIV antibody false positive western blots (WB) and correlation with WB banding pattern. Transfusion 1997;37:1S.
11. Schreiber, GB, Busch, MP, Kleinman, SH, Korelitz, JJ. The risk of transfusion-transmitted viral infections. The Retrovirus Epidemiology Donor Study. N Engl J Med 1996;334:1685-90.
12. Kleinman SH, Busch MP, Korelitz JJ, et al. The incidence/window period model and its use to assess the risk of transfusion-transmitted human immunodeficiency virus and hepatitis C virus infection. Trans Med Rev 1997; 11:155-72.
13. Stramer SL, Porter R, Brodsky JP. Sensitivity of HIV and HCV RNA by pooled genome amplification testing (GAT). Transfusion 1998;38:70S.
14. Busch MP, Korelitz JJ, Kleinman SH, et al. Declining value of alanine aminotransferase in screening of blood donors to prevent posttransfusion hepatitis B and C virus infection. The Retrovirus Epidemiology Donor Study. Transfusion 1995;35:903-10.
15. Aberle-Grasse JM, Dodd RY, Stramer SL. Recent trends in seroprevalence and incidence of HIV-1/2, HCV, and HBV in US allogeneic blood donors. Transfusion 2000;40:5S.
16. Dodd RY, Aberle-Grasse JM, Stramer SL. The yield of nucleic acid testing (NAT) for HIV and HCV RNA in a population of US voluntary donors: relationship to contemporary measures of incidence. Transfusion 2000; 40:1P.

17. Jackson BR, Busch MP, Stramer SL. The cost-effectiveness of nucleic acid testing for HIV, hepatitis C virus and hepatitis B virus in whole blood donations. Submitted for publication.
18. Busch MP, Dodd RY. NAT and blood safety: what is the paradigm? Transfusion 200;40:1157-60.
19. Busch MP, Kleinman SH, Jackson B, et al. Committee report. Nucleic acid amplification testing of blood donors for transfusion-transmitted infectious diseases: Report of the interorganizational task force on nucleic acid amplification testing of blood donors. Transfusion 2000;40:143-59.
20. Roth W, Weber M, Seifried E. Feasibility and efficacy of routine PCR screening of blood donations for hepatitis C virus, hepatitis B virus, and HIV-1 in a blood-bank setting. Lancet 1999;353:359-63.

COST-EFFECTIVENESS OF ALTERNATIVES TO ALLOGENEIC BLOOD TRANSFUSION; REVIEWING THE AVAILABLE EVIDENCE

M. van Hulst[1,2] , Maarten J. Postma[1]

Introduction

Major progress has been made during the last decade in the safety of allogeneic blood products. Donor deferral and extended testing for viruses and bacteria substantially reduced risks associated with blood transfusion. The window period of detection is almost closed and any remaining pathogen might in future be eliminated by pathogen inactivation. However, the small risk of complications after blood transfusion still remains a major concern to the general public and health policy makers. The perception of these risks and potential judicial consequences cause decision makers to favour implementation of procedures to further improve blood transfusion safety [1]. Besides improving safety of allogeinic blood products itself, risk reduction can be achieved by limiting the number of allogeinic transfusions transfused to the recipient. These conservation strategies comprise autologous transfusion, acute normovolemic hemodilution, use of blood growth factors (erythropoietin), peri-operative cell salvage, artificial blood and development of guidelines for minimal use of blood transfusion [2-4]. The utilisation of conservation technologies varies between and within countries [5]. From a pharmaco-economic point of view it is relevant to investigate whether monetary benefits of averted transfusion complications by conservation techniques surpass the costs, or, whether the marginal net costs justify the health gains achieved.

This review investigates the pharmaco-economic evaluations of strategies to enhance blood transfusion safety by lowering the number of units transfused to the recipient. By doing so, this review aims to put the value of conservation techniques in addition to the current safety level into perspective.

In a first step, we provide a brief overview of pharmaco-economic principles and guidelines and discuss the pharmaco-economic aspects of the selected studies. Secondly, we review pharmaco-economic research by type of conservation technique for selected patient groups.

1. Department of Social Pharmacy, Pharmaco-epidemiology and Pharmacotherapy Groningen University Institute for Drug Exploration / University of Groningen Research Institute of Pharmacy (GUIDE / GRIP), Groningen, NL.
2. Department of Clinical Pharmacy and Toxicology, Martini Hospital, Groningen, NL.

Pharmaco-economics

The science of pharmaco-economics has significantly progressed in recent years. Although a lot of disagreement among pharmaco-economists existed in the early nineties, over the recent years more consensus on methodology has been reached [6-8]. This development resulted in a standardised approach, allowing valid comparisons of studies in different fields of health care and across countries [9-12]. The main study types used in economic evaluation are cost-effectiveness (CEA) and cost-utility analysis (CUA) in which the incremental net costs of a programme are related to the incremental health benefits.

CEAs measure health effects in physical units such as increments in life-years gained, infections averted, cases found, cases cured etc. In CUA, the incremental life-years gained are adjusted for quality of life, to arrive at a common measure known as quality adjusted life-year (QALY). Costs are measured in monetary units. Cost-effectiveness or cost-utility ratios are expressed as net costs per unit of effect by comparing the new intervention with current practice (incremental analysis).

Depending on the perspective of a pharmaco-economic evaluation, different types of costs are considered. Generally, all pharmaco-economic analyses include *direct* costs for medical care borne by the health system, community and patient's families. Direct costs can either be *program-related*, such as tests in a screening programme or can be *patient-related*, such as hospital, outpatient and community care. Pharmaco-economic analyses performed from the health care providers' perspective tend to focus on direct costs only. The current consensus in pharmaco-economics is that a more complete model is achieved with the use of a societal perspective and therefore that all relevant costs and consequences for society should be considered, including productivity and leisure losses [13]. However, discussion remains whether loss of productivity caused by morbidity and mortality should be incorporated as *indirect* costs or as quality adjustments in cost-utility analysis [9,11,12,14-16] . Indirect costs may have only a limited impact on pharmaco-economic evaluations of blood transfusion safety, caused by the relatively advanced age of the average transfusion recipient.

Patient-related costs – direct as well as indirect – may transfer to *benefits* if illnesses and related costs are averted, for example through screening or treatment of blood products. The basic concept in pharmaco-economic analyses is to evaluate the net costs, i.e. programme costs minus patient-related benefits. From a pharmaco-economic viewpoint any new programme with negative net cost (offering overall cost saving programs) – and non-negative health gains – should be implemented since it is a dominant strategy. Positive net cost should be related to health gains such as life-years gained. To determine whether implementation is justified, the cost-to-health-gains ratio should be carefully considered and compared to acceptability thresholds, if available.

As viral infections often involve serious complications requiring complex health-care interventions occurring several years after infection, the concept of discounting of future costs is relevant also for transfusion medicine. Examples of long-term complications are cirrhosis after years of chronic hepatitis or development of AIDS in the late stage of HIV-infection. Discounting is a method to adjust future costs and benefits to their present value (cost and benefits are less weighted the farther in the future they accrue). The discounting procedure applies two major principles. Firstly, capital invested in a new technology could have been invested otherwise and may have gained interest. Secondly, there is a pure time preference with short-term benefits being preferred to future with respect to uncertainty as to whether one will be able to benefit from the monetary amount next year as one is now. The value of the discount rate should be chosen in accordance with marginal rates on investment and market interest rates. Many countries use average interest rates of long-term government bonds [15]. Often, discount rates are specified in the national guidelines for pharmaco-economic research and vary between 3% for the USA to 6% for the United Kingdom [13].

Sensitivity analysis is an important tool to investigate the outcomes obtained from pharmaco-economic models. Whereas most parameters used in the models are derived from clinical trials or from retrospective data sources, others may be based on individual expert opinions. Often, few parameters are known with a high degree of undisputed accuracy. To estimate the effect of uncertain variables on the robustness of the model results, sensitivity analysis is performed.

Table 1. Study characteristics and pharmaco-economic aspects of the selected studies

Conservation Technique	**Year**	**Perspective**	**Discounting**		**Risk (per 100,000 units)**		
			Monetary	**Health**	**FTR**	**HIV**	**HCV**
Pre-AD [18]	1993	Hospital	5%	5%	0.2	1	33
Pre-AD [19]	1994	Health Care	5%	5%	0.2	0.65	33
Pre-AD [20]	1995	Health Care	5%	5%	n.s.	0.67	30
IO-AT [21]	1997	Health Care	5%	0%	0.2	0.22	30
PO-AT [22]	1998	Health Care	n.i.	n.i.	n.i.	0.2	0.97
EPO [23]	1998	Health Care	5%	5%	6.3	0.08	0.42
EPO [24]	1998	Health Care	5%	5%	0.16	0.2	1
Pre-AD [25]	1999	Health Care	3%	3%	0.2	0.19	0.97
Pre-AD, EPO [26]	2000	Health Care	5%	5%	6.3	0.08	0.42
PO-AT [27]	2000	Health Care	5%	5%	n.i.	0.15	0.97
EPO [28]	2000	Health Care	5%	5%	0.16	0.2	1

Abbreviations: EPO = erytropoietin; FTR = Fatal Transfusion Reaction ; HCV = Hepatitis C Viru Department of Clinical Pharmacy and Toxicology, Martini Hospital, Groningen, NLs ; HIV = Human Immunodeficiency Virus ; IO-AT = intraoperative autologous transfusion ; n.i. = not included; n.s. = not specified; PO-AT = postoperative autologous transfusion ; Pre-AD = preoperative autologous donation.

Table 2. Cost-utility of autologous transfusion compared to allogeneic transfusion alone (preoperative autologous donations, except where stated).

Patient Group	Year	Additional cost (US$/unit)	Waste (%)	Cost-utility (US$/QALY*)
Cardiac surgery				
CABG [19] †	1994	21	-	508,000-909,000
CABG [20]	1995	107	28	494,000
CABG [26]	2000	63	10	1,785,000
CABG [25]	2000	-	28	3,410,000
CABG [26] (+IM‡)	2000	63	10	cost saving
CABG [25] (+IM)	2000	-	28	1,470
CABG, Valve, Tx (postoperative) [22]	1998	-	-	cost saving
Orthopaedic Surgery				
Bilateral joint replacement [18]	1993	8-33	-	40,000-241,000
Hip replacement [18]	1993	56-73	-	373,000-740,000
Orthopaedic [20]	1995	68	16	235,000
Hip [25]	1999	54	16	3,490,000
Knee replacement [18]	1993	112-139	50	1,147,000-1,467,000
Hip (+IM) [25]	1999	54	16	2,470
Joint arthroplasty (postoperative) [27]	2000	-	-	6,700,000
Miscellaneous Surgery				
Transurethral prostatectomy [20]	1995	4,783	96	23,646,000
Transurethral prostatectomy [25]	1999	54	96	129,000,000
Transurethral prostatectomy (+IM) [25]	1999	54	96	115,000
Abdominal hysterectomy [20]	1995	594	74	1,358,000
Abdominal hysterectomy [25]	1999	54	74	8,930,000
Abdominal hysterectomy (+IM) [25]	1999	54	74	7,333
Abdominal Aortic Aneurysm (intraoperative) [21]	1997	-	-	121,000
AortoIliac Occlusive Disease (intraoperative) [21]	1997	-	-	578,000

* Quality Adjusted Life-Yyear.
† Coronary Artery Bypass Graft.
‡ Immuno Modulation included.

Table 3: Cost-utility of erytropoietin (EPO) in minimising blood transfusion (solely or combined with preoperative autologous donation; pre-AD).

	Year	Patient Group	Cost-utility (US$/QALY*)
EPO + allogeneic versus allogeinic [23]	1998	Cancer Chemotherapy	190,000
EPO versus no intervention [28]	1999	Orthopaedic	48,200,000‡,Ξ
EPO versus no intervention [26]	2000	CABG	7,767,000
EPO versus no intervention(+IM†) [26]	2000	CABG	6,300
Pre-AD + EPO versus no intervention [26]	2000	CABG	5,740,000
Pre-AD + EPO versus no intervention (+IM†) [26]	2000	CABG	cost saving
Pre-AD + EPO versus Pre-AD [26]	2000	CABG	12,600,000
Pre-AD + EPO versus Pre-AD [26]	2000	Cardiac Surgery	31,200,000‡,Ψ
Pre-AD + EPO versus Pre-AD [29]	1999	Orthopaedic	240,200,000‡,Ξ

* Quality Adjusted Life-Year.
† Immuno modulation included.
‡ Per life gained.
Ξ 1 Can$ = 0.7 US$ (1999).
Ψ 1 Can$ = 0.73 US$ (2000).

Study characteristics and pharmaco-economic aspects

We searched MEDLINE for combinations of MESH(sub)-heading "blood transfusion", "cost(-)effectiveness" or "cost(-)utility". We only included full pharmaco-economic evaluations using outcome measures expressed in net cost per life-year or per QALY gained and cost analyses that indicate net cost savings. As outlined above, net cost savings do not necessarily require a full pharmaco-economic analysis, given non-negative health gains. Only studies on alternatives to blood transfusion were included. Studies which expressed cost-effectiveness as costs per allogeneic transfusion avoided were not included.

The MEDLINE search yielded 170 papers. From these 170 studies 11 studies matched our selection criteria. Pre-, peri- and postoperative autologous blood transfusion was the most encountered subject for pharmaco-economic evaluation, in all except one of the selected papers autologous transfusion was evaluated. Minimising allogeinic transfusion by erytropoietine treatment with or without autologous transfusion was evaluated in 4 studies. Major patient groups included in studies were cardiac-, orthopaedic-, urology surgery. Pharmaco-economic evaluations of acute normovolemic hemodilution or adherence to transfusions guidelines - that matched our inclusion criteria - were not found.

All pharmaco-economic simulations used epidemiological data or data obtained from retrospective healthcare databases. Three studies on erytropoietine augmentation of preoperative autologous donations utilised results from clinical randomised trail to establish assumptions [24,26,28]. The perspective of the health care provider was the most utilised viewpoint (10 out of 11). One of the selected papers applied the hospital perspective in the analysis. Univariate and/or multivariate sensitivity analysis was carried out in all evaluations. Health benefits were discounted (3-5%) in 9 of 11 studies and monetary discounting was performed in 10 of 11 evaluations.

The mean age of the blood transfusion recipient was similar for all the analyses and ranged from 60 to 70 years. The risk of HIV, HCV and HBV transmission ranged from 0.08-1, 0.42-33 and 0.5-2 per 100,000 units, respectively.

Autologous transfusion

Autologous transfusion is very appealing to patients and the medical society, because it lowers the chance to be exposed to transfusion of "someone else's" blood with the inherent risks. Because of the risk perception involving allogeneic blood transfusion, a substantial part of surgical patients may choose for autologous transfusion if the procedure is offered to them [29]. Procedures available to reduce allogeneic exposure by transfusing the patients own blood include: preoperative autologous donation with or without erytropoietin augmentation, acute normovolemic hemodilution, intraoperative salvage of blood and postoperative transfusion of shed blood.

The cost-utility of preoperative autologous donations varied from cost saving to US$129 million per QALY gained, see table 2. Considering only viral transmission risks in the economic evaluation cost-utility of preoperative autologous donations in coronary artery bypass graft (CABG) surgery varied from US$0.5 million to US$3.4 million per QALY gained. A range of US$40,000 to US$6.7 million was found for orthopaedic surgery. Preoperative autologous donations in transurethral prostectomy are associated with very unfavourable cost-utility ratios up to US$129,000,000 per QALY gained. An economic evaluation of intra-operative autologous transfusion during elective infrarenal aortic reconstruction revealed cost-utility ratios between US$121,000 to US$578,000 per QALY gained. Postoperative autologous transfusion was shown to be cost saving in cardiac surgery, whereas cost utility ratios for orthopaedic surgery were up to US$6.7 million per QALY gained.

Economic evaluations performed around 1993-1995 showed similar cost-utility ratios for the different patient groups respectively. These utility ratios were lower (i.e. more favourable) compared to cost-utility ratios found after 1999 for the different patient groups. The cost-utility ratios determined from the models strongly depended on the assumed transmission risk of the virus with the highest incidence, i.e. the Hepatitis C virus.

Transfusion requirements in surgery greatly influenced cost-utility of preoperative donation. For instance, in transurethral prostatectomy only about 10% of preoperative donated units are transfused to the patient. This results in cost-utility ratios of US$24 million to US$129 million per QALY gained. Transfusion practices had a considerable impact on the outcome of cost-utility models in preoperative autologous donation. For CABG-surgery patients, the cost-utility of pre-surgery donation of two units changed from well above US$1 million to about US$175,000 per QALY gained for patients of 60 years old in hospitals with low (2,5 units per CABG-patient) and high (5.1 units per CABG-patient) transfusion practices [19].

The models evaluating pre-operative autologous donation assumed in baseline that the autologous procedure itself causes no morbidity and mortality. However, a limited number of case reports on the adverse effects of preoperative autologous donations were published [30]. It was estimated that a fatality rate of above 1 per 103,000 preoperative donations for autologous transfusion in CABG-patients causes health losses to surpass the gains [19].

An increase in postoperative infections associated with or caused by immunomodulation is suggested with allogeneic transfusion [31-35]. Therefore, autologous transfusion could potentially ameliorate the suggested increase in postoperative infections through allogeneic transfusion. When the immunomodulation and associated postoperative infections are included in the economic evaluations of autologous preoperative donation, cost-utility ratios improved from several millions of US$ per QALY gained to a few thousand US$ per QALY gained or even cost saving [25,31].

Erythropoietin

Reduction of exposure to allogeneic transfusion can be also achieved by erythropoietin with or without preoperative autologous donation. Randomised double blind clinical trials indicate that preoperative erytropoietin therapy in combination with iron supplementation is able to reduce exposure to allogeneic transfusion in surgery. No significant reduction of allogeneic transfusion was displayed for erythropoietin 300 or 150 IU/kg starting 5 days before surgery for a total of 8 days compared to placebo (n=182) [36]. However, erythropoietin 5 times 500 IU/kg over fourteen days preoperatively reduced patients requiring transfusion to 11% compared to 53% in the placebo group (n= 76, p=0.0003) in addition to intraoperative isovolemic hemodilution [37]. It is argued that dose of erythropoietin, a prolonged preoperative dosing schedule and the inclusion of an autologous conservation procedure enhances the reduction in allogeneic transfusion [38].

Cost-utility ratios of erythropoietin as a single strategy to minimise allogeneic transfusion were between US$190,000 up to US$48.2 million per QALY gained (see table 3). Erythropoietin treatment used in conjunction with preoperative autologous donation compared to preoperative autologous donation alone yielded cost-utility ratios from US$12.6 million up to US$240million per QALY gained. The cost-utility ratios of erythropoietin in combination with preoperative donation incremental to allogeneic transfusion was estimated at US$5.7 million per QALY gained. When the immunomodulatory effect of allogeneic transfusion was included, cost-utility ratios of erythropoietin based strategies declined. In CABG-patients health gains were surpassed by losses in health if autologous preoperative donation and erythropoietin showed a mortality rate above 1 per 500 [26].

Discussion and conclusion

A wide spectrum of cost-utility ratios was encountered in this review of alternatives for blood transfusion ranging from cost saving for postoperative transfusion of shed mediastinal blood to over hundred million US dollars per QALY gained for preoperative autologous transfusion in transurethral prostectomy and erythropoietin augmentation of preoperative autologous donation in orthopaedic surgery. In general cost-utility ratios of measures to improve blood transfusion safety are strongly influenced by key parameters such as the relatively advanced age of the blood transfusion recipient, increased mortality caused by underlying medical condition and the incubation time of pathogens. Sensitivity analysis included in economic evaluations discussed in this paper showed for instance increasing (worsening) cost-utility ratios with increasing transfusion recipient age.

It appears from the selected studies that cost-utility ratios are rising the last decades. This change towards less value for money and therefore higher cost-utility ratios is probably caused by declining viral transmission risks. All models were sensitive to changes in HCV transmission risks. The halving of the HCV transmission risk assumed in the evaluations between the 1993-1995 period and the period from 1999 onwards increased the cost-utility ratio substantially. Still, the transmission risks assumed in all the economic analysis were substantially higher than recent estimated risks of 0.043 per 100,000 transfusions for HIV and 0.16 for HCV [39]. Therefore, performing an economic re-evaluation with current risk estimates would probably yield even higher cost-utility ratios. Closing the window period of viral screening further by implementation of nucleic acid amplification testing will further increase the cost-utility ratios [40].

The cost-utility ratio of preoperative autologous donation was very sensitive to the actual number of donated unit transfused and thus unused and discarded units. So, low value for money (i.e. high cost-utility ratios) were found for patients with limited transfusion requirements due to discarding of unutilised preoperative donated units.

One evaluation showed postoperative infusion of mediastinal shed blood to be cost saving [22]. This study assumed life-time costs of treating sequelae of relevant viruses and other infection to be equal for all recipients. However, this assumption may overestimate the costs given the incubation time of the viruses in combination with the relatively advanced age of the blood transfusion recipient, in general between 60 to 65 years in cardiac surgery. Furthermore, discounting was neglected in this study further overestimating the potential savings. In orthopaedic surgery postoperative recovery and subsequent transfusion of shed blood displayed a relatively high cost-utility ratio.

Erythropoietin was assumed to reduce the chance of exposure to homologous transfusion in all economic evaluations and therefore avoided allogeneic transfusion related adverse effects. For instance, in elective cardiac surgery with preoperative autologous donation erythropoietin augmentation reduced the number of units transfused from approximately 34% to 58% [24,26]. However, the estimated health gains resulting from the avoidance of blood transfusion were limited and accompanied by high costs involving erythropoietin treatment.

Moreover, adverse effects of erythropoietin treatment cannot be ruled out yet and might increase the cost-utility ratios [36,38].

Transfusion of allogeneic red blood cells is associated with an increased chance of postoperative infections [33-35,41]. Transfusion related immunomodulation (TRIM) could be the underlying mechanism. When this potential effect of blood transfusion is included in economic evaluations the cost-utility significantly improves, because of reduced morbidity and mortality and averted high costs accompanying (postoperative) infections induced by allogeneic blood transfusion. Because TRIM and its role in adverse effects of allogeneic transfusion is still debated, immunomodulatory effects of allogeneic should only be explored in the sensitivity until more definite evidence comes available.

The threshold for pharmaco-economic acceptability has been published at US$50,000 per QALY gained in the USA [42]. However, the pharmacoeconomic acceptance criteria and thresholds differ between health-care settings, societies and interventions. For instance, cost-effectiveness ratios in health care of approximately US$100,000 to US$1,000,000 per life-year gained are readily accepted for transplantation and intensive care settings [43-45]. Cost-effectiveness estimations of injury reducing interventions outside health care also often exceed US$50,000, for example airbags require US$120,000 per life-year saved and seatbelts for school bus passengers costs US$2,800,000 per life-year saved [44]. Furthermore, the USA Federal Aviation Authority uses a threshold of US$2.7 million per life saved for economic acceptability which relates to approximately US$60,000 to US$70,000 per life-year gained for the average air traveller of 35-40 years old [46]. Most of the procedures to minimise allogeneic transfusion did not show cost-utility ratios below the current US$50,000 per QALY gained threshold for economic acceptability.

Up until now alternatives to blood transfusion can't be regarded as cost-effective health care interventions for the general population. In future the balance might shift to cost-effectiveness if adverse effects of allogeneic transfusion such as bacterial infection can be substantiated.

Governed by society's perception of blood transfusion risks [1], governments seem to be willing to allocate significant budgets to improve transfusion safety. However, we have to keep in mind that if health budgets are fixed, allocation of budgets to less favourable cost-effective strategies in health care, neglects potential other more cost-effective strategies with higher health gains.

Acknowledgement

We acknowledge the support of the Landsteiner Foundation for Blood Transfusion Research, grant 0027.

References

1. Finucane ML, Slovic P, Mertz CK. Public perception of the risk of blood transfusion. Transfusion 2000;40:1017-22.
2. Practice strategies for elective red blood cell transfusion. American College of Physicians. Ann Intern Med. 1992;116:403-06.

3. Goodnough LT, Brecher ME, Kanter MH, AuBuchon JP. Transfusion medicine. Second of two parts--blood conservation. N Engl J Med 1999;340:525-33.
4. Practice Guidelines for blood component therapy: A report by the American Society of Anesthesiologists Task Force on Blood Component Therapy. Anesthesiology 1996;84:732-47.
5. Fergusson D, Blair A, Henry D, et al. Technologies to minimize blood transfusion in cardiac and orthopedic surgery. Results of a practice variation survey in nine countries. International Study of Peri-operative Transfusion (ISPOT) Investigators. Int J Technol Assess Health Care 1999;15:717-28.
6. Drummond M, Brandt A, Luce B, Rovira J. Standardizing methodologies for economic evaluation in health care. Practice, problems, and potential. Int J Technol Assess Health Care 1993;9:26-36.
7. Drummond MF, O'Brien B, Stoddart GL, Torrance GW. Methods for the Economic Evaluation of Health Care Programmes. Oxford: Oxford University Press, 1997.
8. Gold MR, Siegel JE, Russel LB, Weinstein MC. Cost-effectiveness in Health and Medicine. New York: Oxford University Press, 1996.
9. Russell LB, Gold MR, Siegel JE, Daniels N, Weinstein MC. The role of cost-effectiveness analysis in health and medicine. Panel on Cost-Effectiveness in Health and Medicine. JAMA 1996;276:1172-77.
10. Siegel JE, Weinstein MC, Russell LB, Gold MR. Recommendations for reporting cost-effectiveness analyses. Panel on Cost-Effectiveness in Health and Medicine. JAMA 1996;276:1339-41.
11. Siegel JE, Torrance GW, Russell LB, Luce BR, Weinstein MC, Gold MR. Guidelines for pharmacoeconomic studies. Recommendations from the panel on cost effectiveness in health and medicine. Panel on cost Effectiveness in Health and Medicine. Pharmacoeconomics. 1997;11:159-68.
12. Weinstein MC, Siegel JE, Gold MR, Kamlet MS, Russell LB. Recommendations of the Panel on Cost-effectiveness in Health and Medicine. JAMA 1996;276:1253-58.
13. Hjelmgren J, Berggren F, Andersson F. Health economic guidelines--similarities, differences and some implications. Value Health 2001;4:225-50.
14. Weinstein MC, Siegel JE, Garber AM, et al. Productivity costs, time costs and health-related quality of life: a response to the Erasmus Group. Health Econ. 1997;6:505-10.
15. Brouwer WB, Koopmanschap MA, Rutten FF. Productivity costs measurement through quality of life? A response to the recommendation of the Washington Panel. Health Econ. 1997;6:253-59.
16. Brouwer WB, Koopmanschap MA, Rutten FF. Productivity costs in cost-effectiveness analysis: numerator or denominator: a further discussion. Health Econ. 1997;6:511-14.
17. Jefferson T, Demicheli V, Mugford M. Elementary Economic Evaluation in Health Care. London: BMJ Publishing Group, 1996.
18. Birkmeyer JD, Goodnough LT, AuBuchon JP, Noordsij PG, Littenberg B. The cost-effectiveness of preoperative autologous blood donation for total hip and knee replacement. Transfusion 1993;33:544-51.

19. Birkmeyer JD, AuBuchon J, Littenberg B, et al. Cost-effectiveness of preoperative autologous donation in coronary artery bypass grafting. Ann Thorac Surg. 1994;57:161-69.
20. Etchason J, Petz L, Keeler E, et al. The cost effectiveness of preoperative autologous blood donations. N Engl J Med. 1995;332:719-24.
21. Huber TS, McGorray SP, Carlton LC, et al. Intraoperative autologous transfusion during elective infrarenal aortic reconstruction: a decision analysis model. J Vasc Surg. 1997;25:984-93.
22. Kilgore ML,.Pacifico AD. Shed mediastinal blood transfusion after cardiac operations: a cost-effectiveness analysis. Ann Thorac Surg. 1998;65:1248-54.
23. Barosi G, Marchetti M, Liberato NL. Cost-effectiveness of recombinant human erythropoietin in the prevention of chemotherapy-induced anaemia. Br J Cancer 1998;78:781-87.
24. Coyle D, Lee KM, Fergusson DA, Laupacis A. Cost effectiveness of epoetin-alpha to augment preoperative autologous blood donation in elective cardiac surgery. Pharmacoeconomics. 2000;18:161-71.
25. Sonnenberg FA, Gregory P, Yomtovian R, et al. The cost-effectiveness of autologous transfusion revisited: implications of an increased risk of bacterial infection with allogeneic transfusion. Transfusion 1999;39:808-17.
26. Marchetti M,.Barosi G. Cost-effectiveness of epoetin and autologous blood donationin reducing allogeneic blood transfusions incoronary artery bypass graft surgery. Transfusion 2000;40:673-81.
27. Jackson BR, Umlas J, AuBuchon J. The cost-effectiveness of postoperative recovery of RBCs in preventing transfusion-associated virus transmission after joint arthtoplasty. Transfusion 2000;40:1063-66.
28. Coyle D, Lee KM, Fergusson DA, Laupacis A. Economic analysis of erythropoietin use in orthopaedic surgery. Transfus Med 1999;9:21-30.
29. Goodnough LT, Monk TG, Brecher ME. Autologous blood procurement in the surgical setting: lessons learned in the last 10 years. Vox Sang 1996;71:133-41.
30. Faught C, Wells P, Fergusson D, Laupacis A. Adverse effects of methods for minimizing perioperative allogeneic transfusion: a critical review of the literature. Transfus Med Rev 1998;12:206-25.
31. Vamvakas EC,.Carven JH. Transfusion and postoperative pneumonia in coronary artery bypass graft surgery: effect of the length of storage of transfused red cells. Transfusion 1999;39:701-10.
32. Vamvakas EC,.Carven JH. Length of storage of transfused red cells and postoperative morbidity in patients undergoing coronary artery bypass graft surgery. Transfusion 2000;40:101-09.
33. Vamvakas EC,.Blajchman MA. Deleterious clinical effects of transfusion-associated immunomodulation: fact or fiction? Blood 2001;97:1180-95.
34. Leal-Noval SR, Rincon-Ferrari MD, Garcia-Curiel A, Herruzo-Aviles A, Camacho-Larana P, Garnacho-Montero J et al. Transfusion of blood components and postoperative infection in patients undergoing cardiac surgery. Chest 2001;119:1461-68.

35. Chelemer SB, Prato BS, Cox PM, Jr., O'Connor GT, Morton JR. Association of bacterial infection and red blood cell transfusion after coronary artery bypass surgery. Ann Thorac Surg 2002;73:138-42.
36. D'Ambra MN, Gray RJ, Hillman R, et al. Effect of recombinant human erythropoietin on transfusion risk in coronary bypass patients. Ann Thorac Surg 1997;64:1686-93.
37. Sowade O, Warnke H, Scigalla P, et al. Avoidance of allogeneic blood transfusions by treatment with epoetin beta (recombinant human erythropoietin) in patients undergoing open- heart surgery. Blood 1997;89:411-18.
38. Goodnough LT, Despotis GJ, Parvin CA. Erythropoietin therapy in patients undergoing cardiac operations. Ann.Thorac.Surg. 1997;64:1579-80.
39. Muller-Breitkreutz K. Results of viral marker screening of unpaid blood donations and probability of window period donations in 1997. EPFA Working Group on Quality Assurance. Vox Sang. 2000;78:149-57.
40. Loubiere S, Rotily M, Durand-Zaleski I, Costagliola D. Including polymerase chain reaction in screening for hepatitis C virus RNA in blood donations is not cost-effective. Vox Sang. 2001;80:199-204.
41. Pereira A. Deleterious consequences of allogenic blood transfusion on postoperative infection: really a transfusion-related immunomodulation effect? Blood 2001;98:498-500.
42. Owens DK. Interpretation of cost-effectiveness analyses. J Gen Intern Med 1998;13:716-17.
43. Michel BC, van Hout BA, Bonsel GJ. Assessing the benefits of transplant services. Baillieres Clin Gastroenterol 1994;8:411-23.
44. Tengs TO, Adams ME, Pliskin JS, et al. Five-hundred life-saving interventions and their cost-effectiveness. Risk Anal 1995;15:369-90.
45. Al MJ, Koopmanschap MA, van Enckevort PJ, Geertsma A, et al. Cost-effectiveness of lung transplantation in The Netherlands: a scenario analysis. Chest 1998;113:124-30.
46. Hoffer S, Berardino F, Smith J, Rubin S. Economic Values for Evaluation of FAA Investment and Regulatory Decisions. Washington, DC: Federal Aviation Administration, Office of Aviation Policy, Plans, and Management Analysis Publication FAA-APO-98-8, 1998.

HEREDITARY METABOLIC DISEASES AND STEM CELL TRANSPLANTATION.

G. Peter A. Smit[1]

Introduction

The majority of metabolic diseases is transmitted in the autosomal recessive mode. In this publication metabolic diseases following this mode of transmission will be discussed. For reasons of simplification these metabolic diseases are divided in bone marrow related (BR) and non-bone marrow related (non-BR). In the bone marrow related metabolic diseases the biochemical defect is expressed within the bone marrow resulting in bone marrow disease and ultimately in progressive bone abnormalities.

Two aspects will be discussed: hereditary metabolic diseases and donor suitability, and hereditary metabolic diseases and therapeutic bone marrow (stem cell) transplantation (BMT/SCT).

Hereditary metabolic diseases and donor suitability

The present practice in The Netherlands in the judgement of donor suitability with respect to metabolic diseases in relatives in the first degree (biological father, mother, other siblings) is that this potent donor is not accepted. In case of non-BR metabolic diseases, even when the potent donor is homozygous for the disease, this is an unnecessary measure because these genetic diseases will not be expressed in bone marrow. In the – hypothetical – situation that the bone marrow-derived stem cells, after migration, will be expressed in other tissues, the normal enzyme activity in the subsequent organs of the recipient will be able to correct for the expected small accumulation of pre-enzyme substrates. For example in the case of a donor with a disorder of amino acid, carbohydrate, or fatty acid metabolism the hypothetical accumulation of pre-enzyme metabolites will be rapidly metabolised by the normal liver enzymes of the recipient.

When the donor is heterozygous for the non-BR metabolic disease there are no contra-indications whatsoever from a metabolic point of view [1,2]. In case of BR metabolic diseases when the potent donor is homozygous for the metabolic disease the donor is not acceptable because the disease will be expressed in bone marrow and cause bone marrow and bone disease. When the potentential donor is heterozygous for the BR metabolic disease no abnormalities are

1. Department of Metabolic Diseases, Beatrix Children's Hospital University Hospital Groningen, NL.

expected from a metabolic point of view. A less strict strategy in case of potent donors with metabolic diseases is advocated.

Hereditary metabolic diseases and therapeutic bone marrow (stem cell) transplantation

BMT/SCT is applied in patients with BR metabolic diseases, especially the lysosomal storage diseases [1-3]. The prevalence of the lysosomal diseases in The Netherlands is twice as high as PKU (phenylketonuria) or MCADD (medium chain acetyl-CoA dehydrogenase deficiency) and represents therefore a considerable medical problem for society [4]. Within the scope of enzyme replacement therapy BMT has been performed in these diseases for many years. Due to many factors the results of this therapy were not very favourable. The difficulty of the replaced enzyme in the crossing of the blood-brain-barrier in the lysosomal diseases with CNS involvement for example is an important complication. The poor response of the bone abnormalities is another major drawback. Moreover, both morbidity and mortality are significantly higher after BMT in lysosomal diseases. One of the reasons is the higher incidence of graft rejection [2,3]. BMT/SCT is regarded not a cure for the metabolic patients, but may improve the quality of life.

In general, if applied, BMT/SCT should be performed in children with the more gradual evolving variants, especially before neurological abnormalities are present [1-3]. In this case the potent donor should not be heterozygous for the underlying metabolic disorder.

Future expectations

The poor results after BMT in lysosomal storage diseases might be improved by using bone marrow-derived mesenchymal stem cells instead. Mesenchymal stem cells have the potency not only to migrate to non-haematopoietic tissues (and even cross the blood-brain-barrier), but also to transform into other cells of mesenchymal origin [5]. The development of the use of bone marrow derived mesenchymal stem cells as targets for gene therapy seems promising. Important problems that remain are the persistence of expression of enzyme production and the lack of convenient neurotropic vectors [6,7]. In view of the latter the potential role of newly developed inhibitors of synthesis of the substrate of the deficient enzyme may well be an important new therapeutic strategy. These inhibitors are derived from imino sugars and because of their simple structure able to cross the blood-brain-barrier [8].

References

1. Beck M. Mucopolysaccharides and Oligosaccharides. In: Fernandes J, Saudubray .M, van den Berghe G (eds), Inborn Metabolic Diseases, Diagnosis and Treatment. Springer Verlag ISBN 3-540-65626. Third edition, 2001.
2. Steward CG. Bone marrow transplantation for genetic diseases. In: Fairbarn LJ, Testa NG (eds) Blood cell Biochemistry. Volume 8: Haemopoiesis and Gene Therapy. New York: Kluwer Academic/Plenum Publishers. 13-56.

3. Wraith JE. Advances in the treatment of lysosomal storage disease. Dev Med Child Neurol 2001;43:639-46.
4. Poorthuis BJ, Wevers RA, KLeijer WJ, et al. The frequency of lysosomal storage disease in The Netherlands. Human Genetics 1999;105:151-56.
5. Koç ON, Peters Ch, Augbourg P, et al.. Bone marrow-derived mesenchymal stem cells remain host-derived despite successful hematopoietic engraftment after allogenic transplantation in patients with lysosomal and peroxysomal storage diseases. Exp Hematol 1999;27:1675-81.
6. Schumann EH. Hematopoietic stem cell gene therapy for Niemann-Pick disease and other lysosomal storage diseases. Chem Phys Lipids 1999;102: 179-88.
7. Baxter MA, Wynn RF, Deakin JA, et al. Retrovirally mediated correction of bone marrow-derived mesenchymal stem cells from patients with muco-polysaccharidosis type I. Blood 2002;99:1857-59.
8. Platt FM, Jeyakumar M, Andersson U, Priestmann DA, Dwek RA, Butters TD. Inhibition of substrate synthesis as a strategy for glycolipid lysosomal storage disease therapy. J Inher Metab Dis 2001;24:275-90.

DETECTION OF DISEASE: POSSIBILITIES AND LIMITATIONS

Joost Th.M. de Wolf[1]

Introduction

Much has and can be done to make blood transfusion as safe as possible. These include preventive measures beginning with donor education, screening, selection and deferral procedures, post-donation product quarantine and donor tracing when transmission of an infectious agent occurred. In addition we can test the blood for the presence of infectious agents. We can also use inactivation methods like solvent and detergent, or replace the use of blood by alternatives such as recombinant products, for instance clotting factor VIII or IX or the use of blood substitutes. In this paper we will further focus on the screening of blood for infectious agents. At the end it will be clear that blood safety is not equal to the detection of an infectious agent. In order to come as close as possible to the detection of disease the decision to screen for infectious agents should be based on certain principles which will be discussed later.

Problems to face

What kind of problems can we face when we talk about the relation between an infectious agent and disease. There are agents, always leading to disease and sometimes fatal. Other agents are not related to disease at all. Some agents cause disease only when transfused with a minimum dose. Some agents are only related to disease when certain patient characteristics are present. The clinical effects and natural history of HIV infection are known and we know what kind of disease might be prevented by measurements ranging from donor education to serologic testing. There were times that the chance of HIV transmission was about 1.2 in 100; with donor education, screening and selection an effective reduction in the transmission of the infectious agent to 1 in 500 was realized [1].

If an infectious agent like hepatitis C virus is detected in a blood donor, what does it mean for the outcome after transmission, what is the natural history, how serious is it. The Irish Hepatology Research group reported a 17 year follow up of women who had received Rh immunoglobulin contaminated with HCV. Almost 20 years after exposure 314 of 704 infected women demonstrated only anti-HCV without detectable HCV RNA, meaning that 45% of the women demonstrated spontaneous recovery from the infection. ALT values were normal in

1. Dept of Haematology, University Hospital, Groningen, NL.

45% of the women, slightly abnormal in 47% and 8% demonstrated moderately abnormal values. In liver biopsy, fibrosis was absent in 49% of the cases, and cirrhosis was observed in 2% of the women. Two of these 7 women with cirrhosis were heavy drinkers [2]. These figures contrast with the 20% cirrhosis usually reported 20 years after HCV infections. Several variables have been suggested to influence the progression of HCV. Such as the mode of transmission, excessive alcohol intake, HBV and HIV infection, older age at infection and immune host factors [3].

Not all viruses are related to disease. Recently viruses are described which are transmitted by blood in which the clinical relevance is not clear at all.

In 1997 a group of Japanese researchers discovered a new virus, called TT virus (TTV), after the initials of the first patient in whose blood it was initially identified [4]. TTV is a small, non-enveloped virus with a single stranded circular DNA genome. TTV may be related to the Circoviridae, a group of viruses that are known to infect plants and vertebrates, especially swine and birds; chicken anemia virus is the best-characterized member of this family. Although the virus was originally isolated from a patient with transfusion transmitted hepatitis, on the basis of limited published prevalence studies, the association between TTV infection and human hepatitis is questionable.

Dependent on the primers used TTV viremia was detected by PCR (polymerase chain reaction) in blood donors in 1-80% of the cases; in African populations without any identified parenteral exposure in 7-83%, in multitransfused patients in 27% and in IV drug users in 6-40% [5,6]. Recently, the incidence of TTV in 150 transfused patients undergoing a coronary artery bypass graft surgery was reported [7]. 34% of the 137 previously uninfected patients developed new TTV viremia after transfusion. 38 were infected with TTV alone, 5 were co-infected with HGV and 3 with HCV.

In all publications TTV positive patients were mostly asymptomatic; if TTV was associated with chronic liver disease the patient wėre invariably co-infected with either the hepatitis B or C virus. Besides, TTV does not aggravate the symptoms associated with hepatitis B or C; it does not cause post-hepatitis aplastic anemia. The current data did not support an association of TTV infection with liver disease or other pathologic conditions, suggesting that there is no need for systemic detection of TTV infection before blood donation.

The hepatitis G virus was detected in 1996 in a patient with chronic non-A through E hepatitis, and at the same time in another African patient with an acute non-A through E hepatitis [8]. HGV is a lipid enveloped, single stranded RNA virus belonging to the Flavi viridae family, like the HCV. HGV might be detected in plasma or serum by PCR assay or with an antibody assay. This last assay detects antibody to an HGV envelope protein, E_2. Anti-E_2 is a marker that appears when the host successfully clears HGV infection. The prevalence of HGV RNA is 1-4%, whereas the rates of anti-E_2, indicating resolved HGV infection, ranges from 3-14%. The incidence of infection after transfusion is 9.8%, but in heavily transfused patients such as thalassemics or liver transplant recipients the incidence ranges from 20-30%. HGV infections occurs more frequently in HCV-infected persons, indicating common modes of transmission. Numerous well designed controlled studies documented that HGV does not cause any form of liver disease or other types of disease not even in immunosuppressed populations. However there are several case reports and small studies suggesting a possible association of HGV and disease. Because HGV is common in the general population a small percentage of patients might be coincidentally be infected with HGV, and might be seen as an innocent bystander. In general it is impossible to prove that an infectious agent, like HGV, does not cause or contribute to disease; but looking at the evidence we must conclude that if HGV does cause disease of the liver or other organ system, it does so only in a very small number of infected persons. So, although there is a possibility to screen the population before blood donation for HGV with PCR it seems not warrented.

Another question about infectious agents and disease is how many copies of an infectious agent are necessary to induce disease? In other words are there donors with a positive test who are not infectious? Recently, the effects of intravenously inoculation of three chimpanzees with plasma and mononuclear cells of patients who were HBV DNA PCR positive but HBsAg negative were described [9]. None of the animals inoculated developed any evidence of HBV infection. The animals did not develop HBsAg, anti-HBc, ALT abnormalities, or HBV DNA detectable by the quantitative PCR assay, during a follow up for 15 months.

On the other hand blood, HIV negative in the NAT assay was responsible for HIV infection in a platelet recipient and red blood cell recipient. Additional testing using donor screening NAT assays showed consistent detection of HIV RNA in the undiluted donor plasma whereas detection was inconsistent at the 1:16 and 1:24 dilution levels currently used in minipool screening of blood donations in the USA [10].

It is clear that detection of an infectious agent is not the same as detection of disease. In order to come as close as possible to detection of disease, or clinically relevant screening of blood, the decision to screen the blood supply for an infectious agent should be based on scientific evidence that indicates that sufficient benefit is obtained for the recipient. One needs to show that the infectious agent is transfusion-transmitted, that the infectious agent leads to disease in the recipient and what the natural history of the disease is, how many patients are affected, and how serious the disease is.

Possibilities and limitations

Detection of disease

Possibilities and limitations. What have we gained and should new possibilities be implemented or are the limits reached? The risk for HIV infection is reduced from 1 in 100 units to approximately 1 in 680,000 units. The transfusion related hepatitis has also almost been vanquished: the transmission rates for hepatitis C has decreased from 1 in 200 units to 1 in 100,000 units today, and the risk for hepatitis B infection has been reduced from 1 in 2100 to 1 in 63,000. According to the Centers for Disease control and Prevention 40 patients have developed the acquired immunodeficiency syndrome after receiving a transfusion in the united states in the 15 years that blood has been screened for HIV.

Despite the dramatic improvement in blood safety and the low risk of viral transmission, substantial effort and resources continue to be expended to eliminate the few transmissions that remain [11].

The major concern has been donations during the interval between infection and seroconversion, the 'window period' of infection involving donors who are infected but test negative by standard serological screening techniques. A solution is the introduction of methods of direct viral detection using nucleic acid amplification tests (NAT) for HIV, HCV and HBV or for HIV p24 antigen testing.

By testing minipools of 16 to 24 plasma samples 16.3 million donations are tested for HCV RNA and 12.6 million for HIV RNA. 1 in 3.2 million serologically negative donations was positive for HIV RNA, 1 in 263,000 units was positive for HCV RNA [12]. For our hospital which is one of the largest in the Netherlands this would mean 1 clinically important HCV infection in 30 years. If single unit testing instead of minipool testing will be the standard, 1 in 4 million minipool negative donations will be HIV positive, and 1 in 1 million HCV minipool negative donations will be HCV positive. This low yield will be obtained at high costs, for minipool NAT the cost per case detected is estimated at \$1.7 million and \$2.7 million dollars for a case detected by single unit NAT [12].

Detection of disease

Possibilities and limitations. Despite all the possibilities, limits are reached. It may be wiser to look at other problems concerning the safety of blood transfusion and especially problems due to the transfusion of incorrect blood. From the results obtained by the hemovigilance system in the United Kingdom it became clear that the transfusion of incorrect blood is a major problem: 34% of the major morbidity or mortality due to transfusion is caused by errors: patients are not getting the right product [13]. Although it is a problem not easy to attack, it is worth to develop possibilities and hopefully we might conclude in the near future that here to the limits are reached.

References

1. Busch MP, Young MJ, Samson SM, Mosley JW, Ward JW, Perkins HA. Risk of human immunodeficiency virus (HIV) transmission by blood transfusion before the implementation of HIV-1 antibody screening. The Transfusion Safety Study Group. Transfusion 1991;31:4-11
2. Kenny-Walsh E, the Irish hepatology research group. Clinical outcomes after hepatitis C infection from contaminated anti-D immune globulin. N Engl J M 1999;340:1228-33
3. Roudot-Thoraval F, Bastie A, Pawlotsky JM, Dhumeaux D, study group for the prevalence and the epidemiology of hepatitis C virus. Epidemiological factors affecting the severity of hepatitis C virus related liver-disease: a french survey of 6664 patients. Hepatology 1997;26:485-90
4. Nishizawa T, Okamoto H, Konishi K, Yoshizawa H, Miyakawa Y, Mayumi M. A novel DNA virus (TTV) associated with elevated transaminase levels

in posttransfusion hepatitis of unknown etiology. Biochem Biophys Res Comm 1997;241:92-97
5. Handa A, Dickstein B, Young NS, Brown KE. Prevalence of the newly described human circovirus, TTV, in United States blood donors. Transfusion 2000;40:245-52
6. Biagini P, Gallian P, Touinssi M, et al. High prevalence of TT virus infection in French blood donors revealed by the use of three PCR systems. Transfusion 2000;40:590-96
7. Wang JT, Lee CZ, Kao JH, Sheu JC, Wang TH, Chen DS. Incidence and clinical presentation of posttransfusion TT virus infection in prospectively followed transfusion recipients: emphasis on its relevance to hepatitis. Transfusion 2000;40:596-602
8. Kleinman S. Hepatitis G virus biology, epidemiology, and clinical manifestations: implications for blood safety. Transf Med Rev 2001;15:201-13
9. Prince AM, Lee D-H, Brotman B. Infectivity of blood from pcr-positive, HBsAg-negative, anti-HBs-positive cases of resolved hepatitis B infection. Transfusion 2001;41:329-32
10. Ling AE, Robbins KE, Brown TM, et al. Failure of routine HIV-1 tests in a case involving transmission with seroconversion blood components during the infectious window period. JAMA 2000;284:210-14
11. Klein HG. Will blood transfusion ever be safe enough? JAMA 2000;284: 238-40
12. Busch MP and Dodd RY. NAT and blood safety: what is the paradigm? Transfusion 2000;40:1157-60
13. Williamson L, Cohen H, Love E, Jones H, Todd A, Soldan K. The serious hazards of transfusion (SHOT) initiative: the UK approach to haemovigilance. Vox Sang 2000;78 (Suppl 2):291-95.

DISCUSSION

Moderators: D.S. Wages and J.H. Marcelis

C.L. van der Poel (Amsterdam, NL): As a scientist I am not so used to having guidelines on how to perform my science. I understand that the mathematics that you are doing is quite scientific, but I am very curious about guidelines. I understand we have guidelines in the Netherlands and you once told me that there are about 19 regulations you have to fulfil; are the Dutch guidelines then different from the United States? Apparently a life here is differently paid in the United States than in the Netherlands; if so, that is a political decision. But what is the impact of guidelines on these sort of calculations, could you comment on that?

M.J. Postma (Groningen, NL): I agree with you that from a scientific point of view guidelines are very annoying. There was a need for guidelines because the industry is doing a lot of the pharma-economic research themselves. You are able to manipulate your product in the good direction by taking the discount rate that you want or including or excluding medical costs in life-years gained. To avoid this possibility of these studies being completely incomparable these guidelines were developed. It is annoying but sometimes it is easy as well. I mean we have a nice booklet with reference prices for instance, which is sometimes very convenient.

C.L. van der Poel: Are they different in different countries?

M.J. Postma: With respect to the guidelines there are some differences between countries. They – for example – relate to the exact level of the discount rate, but also to more and more relevant choices like taking the friction costing approach or the human capital approach, or whether to include medical costs in life-years gained or not. So, there are some differences.

C.L. van der Poel: Not only on the money but also on the methodology you would have to be very careful to compare data between countries, then?

M.J. Postma: That is true. So, the way I did it in the last part of my talk is a bit crude in that sense.

D.S. Wages (Concord, CA, USA): I have a follow-up question that maybe is a sensible one. Probably other people have this question too. How was the guideline of 20,000 EURO per QALY arrived at? You mentioned it and it might have something to do with cholesterol levels, but who makes that decision and how is that arrived at?

M.J. Postma: It was specifically developed for cholesterol treatment. So, that is why I always doubt if it is of very high relevance for other areas as well. How exactly this choice was made maybe has to do with economical impact, how much money in total you want to spend on the topic. The obvious implication of that is: It is better to treat a non-smoking woman because she has a better prospect of survival than – for example – a male.

R.Y. Dodd (Rockville, MD, USA): Your conclusions about leukocyte depletion were very interesting, but they were very specific to that study I believe. A little earlier this year in Paris Sunny Dzik[1] reported on a study in which he had randomized patients in a hospital over a certain amount of time. He found essentially no cost differential between recipients of routine products and recipients of leukocyte reduced products – it is not cost effectiveness. This was no cost differential in terms of the cost of the therapy of these patients whether or not they received leukocyte reduced blood. You have any comment on that?

M.J. Postma: Just one question. I do not know the details of this study, but did he look into the health effect as well?

R.Y. Dodd: I do not remember fully there are people in the audience that remember better than I do, but I think the issue was really hospital billing – how much the treatment costs. So, there was consideration of immediate health effects in terms of whether the individuals remained longer in hospital and the amount of antibiotics they received.

M.J. Postma: In the data that I am analyzing one of the main drivers of the outcomes is the difference in mortality between the two groups and the effects on the life-years gained; that is clear.

C.L. van der Poel I remember some of that study. There were two arms, about 1300 patients in each arm. They were randomized not according to patient group but all patients receiving blood. So, there was no obvious clinical relevant outcome of that study, because with a mixed patient group you do not get any statistical solid difference in outcome. What was funny though was the total cost of staying in the hospital including all therapies used – that was a primary outcome of the two arms. I have never seen any study were a randomized controlled trial used the total hospital bill as a primary outcome. Because, now we do it very complicated. We first look into cost effectiveness after a clinical study and then translate the cost effectiveness into the real costs. That one could measure the real costs, by looking at the total bill, was new to me.

---

1. Dzik S, Anderson J, O Neill M, Assmann S, Stowell C. Prospective randomized controlled clinical trial of universal leukoreduction. Transf Clin Biol 2001;8 (Suppl 1): 35s-abstract S22-002.

J.H. Marcelis (Tilburg, NL): Dr. Smit, is it thinkable to transduce a hereditary disorder in children who you gave bone marrow transplantation after leukemia for instance and can you introduce such in next generations? We hope that we come as far as that children after bone marrow transplantation become fertile and have offspring. But when you can introduce hereditary diseases this way into the germ cells, would that be thinkable?

G.P.A. Smit (Groningen, NL): I do not know that. I do not think so. Probably your audience is better able to answer that question than I am. Let us say the genetic information should spread into the germ cells and I am not sure that this is the case. But if it were the case, is that harmful to future generations. I mean if you look at for example at phenylketonuria. We all know that in heterozygotes the prevalence or the incidence is one in fifty. If you would transplant one patient with leukemia, with bone marrow from someone who let us assume turns out to be a phenylketonuria patient, how much would you increase the risk in terms of genetic risks in the whole population with that?

J.H. Marcelis: That is a very difficult question.

G.P.A. Smit: I do not know. There is no science.

That is the reason why my opinion is donors, potent donors, are quite acceptable for using bone marrow transplantation in oncology patients.

D.S. Wages: We had four very good talks covering a wide range of issues. Dr. Susan Stramer with her update of NAT testing and her review of what is happening in the United States, Dr. Maarten Postma reviewing the cost of a variety of safety measures, Dr. Peter Smit who reviewed hereditary metabolic diseases and how that can have implications for blood transfusions and finally Dr. Joost de Wolf who reviewed the possibilities for detection of disease for transfusion and anti-transfusion safety. So, are there any questions for these speakers?

C.Th. Smit Sibinga: Dr. Stramer and Dr. de Wolf – two presentations; the first and last one in this session. Dr. Stramer told us where we are today. Dr. de Wolf told us we have reached the limit. What is your opinion?

S.L. Stramer (Gaitherburg, MD, USA): I was just commenting that we all shared a very common theme in that we're detecting less and it is costing us a lot more. I don't know where we are actually going to end considering the cost of NAT testing. For the benefit we are seeing from NAT we could even discuss whether we need to continue to do NAT testing. Additionally, there is the discussion of whether will we ever go to single donation testing. From your data I would say it will take you 60 years to find additional positives beyond mini-pool NAT. So, I think we are at the limit now, at least for HIV, HCV and likely HBV with a good HBsAg test. But I do not know if the lawyers or the regulators in society will take us further. I would say we are where we need to be now with mini-pool testing.

J.Th.M. de Wolf (Groningen, NL): I agree with that, but there are always people who would say: 'When I have a test and I do not use it, what will happen'. I do not have an answer, but I think that for doctors it is completely ridiculous to spend so much money on so little improvement. We are now talking with the government about hemovigilance and that is a very difficult problem. We are asking support for ten nurses in the whole Netherlands to support us. And we are talking about that already for two years. That is for one year one million guilders, but when there comes a new test twenty million guilders do not seem to be a problem. I think that other problems can be solved at less costs. For me it is not understandable that there is such a difference.

S.L. Stramer: The unit of blood is indeed safe. We spend so much emphasis on that unit instead of on the processes around the use of the unit or what happens in the hospital, such as linkage of the donor with the right unit before transfusion. We need to focus less on the product and really look more to the process.

H.J.C. de Wit (Amsterdam, NL): Perhaps I might add to this. I am afraid that we have to consider each test apart, because for the NAT testing now we have two years of experience. For me it is quite clear – continuing NAT testing in minipools is not because of lawyers or product liability, not because we can make an easy calculation that it would be cheaper for the organization not to do it. This discussion is even becoming heavier now that we run into paternalistic discussions which will make this testing even more costly. The problem here is regulators. The solution is perhaps in the EU Directive on blood – common standards and a co-ordinated European discussion about what to do and what not to do. I hope that this discussion can be held very well and co-ordinated on a scientific base, so that not country by country but as a whole we can take decisions what to do and what not to do. But I agree that after two years of NAT testing we can conclude that the added value in our situation is extremely small. So, prioritize and do other things. Other examples that were illustrated by Dr. Postma – bacterial contamination control of platelets – is cost effective in his model and in our situation. I was very pleased to hear that, because we are in the course of introducing such measure. Regarding the environment I would say it is not different clients – doctors are not the only clients we have although that would make life a lot easier because there would be only one group to discuss these things with. But we also have to take into account regulators, the politicians and the public. That makes it complicated and makes decision making for every issue different.

D.S. Wages Dr. de Wolf in your experience you mentioned how the data showed that the added gain for all this additional testing is added all in minimal amounts to the overall safety of the blood supply. But when you talk to your patients what is your perception of their understanding of the risk of transfusion. Do you think that their perception is what leads to a lot of the pressures on regulatory agencies to keep adding additional safety aspects to a correct transfusion medicine practice?

J.Th.M. de Wolf: My patients are hematology and oncology patients and that is no problem at all. I have never had one patient nor in my department nor at the anesthesiology who asked whether it does matter at all if a test results in one in 400,000 positive and another test one in 450,000 positive. If you would use a NAT test for HCV that means that there is residual risk of one HCV infection in a thirty years or less, well I do not think that the patient is waiting for that. Maybe he is waiting for other things you can do with so many millions of dollars.

J.A. van der Does (Den Haag, NL): Dr. de Wolf, I think there is one exception – that is a group of patients called hemophiliacs, who are very focal in the discussion on the political and societal side, very good and know exactly what all the chances are.

I agree with you that the patients receiving some units of platelets or some units of erythrocytes have other things to occupy their minds with.

J.Th.M. de Wolf: Yes, it is a difficult point to talk about hemophiliacs, because they have a dramatic history. That is for sure, but I still think that the problems we have when we talk with hemophiliacs about plasma derived or recombinant products, is it necessary to explain what is the benefit for the patient. That is a difficult discussion, because it is very emotional to talk about that. I have the impression that the same emotions play a role when we are talking or the blood bank is talking with politicians or regulators. That is why I think that it is very important that if you are introducing a new test that you require the scientific evidence about the benefit for patients and our society.

S.L. Stramer: So, the manufacturers at least in the United States are going to force hepatitis B NAT into our cocktail of HIV and HCV NAT, although there is no clinical evidence of posttransfusion hepatitis B even though we do not yet have the most sensitive HBsAg tests in the US. There is no clinical evidence that we need anything else. It is going to be driven by the marketing because the test is there not because the need is there.

H.T.M. Cuypers (Amsterdam, NL): Another problem is history, because this HIV testing started with a major incident. A number of people were infected with an intravenous immunoglobulin preparation. The authorities reacted to this problem and forced manufacturers to do these tests. Since the mid nineties patients are protected from having infected immunoglobulin preparations by doing these NAT testing. However, the problem always is once started, it is difficult to stop the train. Than it comes into regulations and officially accepted which makes it hard to stop. You see with all these tests, the problem is not the decision, it is always a triggering incident starting with something to do and than the possibility to not being able to stop the train anymore.

C.Th. Smit Sibinga: Another issue that was raised – Dr. Stramer started and Dr. Postma followed it up extensively in his presentation on the pharmacoeconometry – is on quality adjustment of life-years. Dr. Postma, to what extent actually do you have indicators for the adjustment of quality; and how have we defined quality; is that a factor that you translate in the costing; and how do you translate that in the costing.

M.J. Postma: There is a difference between Europe, maybe the Netherlands in particular and the USA. In the USA everything is expressed in quality adjusted life-years (QALY) that is gained. Here, at the moment we look at life-years gained often without the quality aspect. There are, however, quality factors available for a lot of health state stages measured in Dutch patients. So, it could be factored in here as well. Whether it will improve or worsen the cost effectiveness that is difficult to say. It can go both ways, but I think at the moment cost per life you gained is what the Dutch Minister of Public Health wants.

C.Th. Smit Sibinga: But the point is – back to the hemophilia patients – do we really have an idea of what the expectations of the consumers are about this gain in life-years and the adjustment of quality before we bring it into our calculation. It is necessary to do it, but this is a question, which we have to relate to the regulations and the enforcement of new tests to come in our armamentarium, assuming that the consumers really expect a better outcome. So far I have not traced much evidence that that is really part of the equation.

M.J. Postma: It is difficult to answer your question except that I heard Dr. de Wolf just saying that he has the idea that the patient may not be so very anxious to get this level of security but that is all I can say at the moment.

J.H. Marcelis: Dr. Smit also talked about the quality of life which should be better after treatment with bone transplants and I wonder if he also has quantitative information about this quality of life.

G.P.A. Smit: I do not have any information on that part, I am sorry and I do not know it from the literature as well.

A follow-up question for dr. Postma. I am very eager to know how the cost per QALY are calculated; I mean Dr Stramer from the US showed us 50,000 dollars and in Canada something like 30,000 dollars or so and we talk about 20,000 € per QALY. It is very difficult to estimate that, especially being a pediatrician. For example we are going to screen for a metabolic disease in the northern part of the Netherlands and we also now need a cost effectiveness study in this screening study. We screen for a metabolic disease that if you miss it the child will die. At the moment we screen for phenylketonuria. If you screen for phenylketonuria and you miss a patient, you will have a patient institutionalized for his whole life where life expectancy in years is normal. So, that will cost a lot of money. The metabolic disease we are going to screen for is one of which the patient will die if you miss it. So, you tell me how to calculate the costs before we burn our hands.

M.J. Postma: All the things you just mentioned – the life long costs and the patients dying, life years lost, it will all be included in the cost effectiveness analysis. Be it per QALY, be it per life-year gained it should all be factored in although there are some type of costs according to the guidelines that should not be included. Than you come up with a figure above or below 20,000 € per life-year gained. We had this discussion after my talk very shortly how did we arrive at the 20,000 €. The feeling is that it is derived from acceptable budgets for cholesterol treatment. There is a budget for cholesterol implicitly in the heads of the decision makers and this budget is optimally distributed to render as much health gains as possible. Some patient groups fall out because they are too old and smokers. I think for Meningococcus C vaccination as an example, totally other acceptable costs per life-year gained would be present in the head of decision-makers.

G.P.A. Smit: For example how much?

M.J. Postma: I do not dare to say.

G.P.A. Smit: Is it less?

M.J. Postma: No, I would not say it is less, no; I think the other way.

S.L. Stramer: I just want to make a point. The test phenylketonuria is very inexpensive, I would imagine. The medical necessity is very high and is driven by a medical need not by the technology. However, in the absence of a medical need and because there is a hepatitis C patent – you know one company owns the sequence to the agent – anyone now doing hepatitis C testing can be forced to pay per donation, because we do pool testing. So, if you are doing a pool of 96 it is 96 times more costs than you have been using for 2 years, because now they are catching you with the patent. We are looking on one extreme end of the scale. I do not know if you could associate the cost the way you described it.

G.P.A. Smit: OK, that is the cost for the screening, but let us say the quality of life also has to do with the morbidity of the patients and the cost of that. Those are probably comparable. So, I was very surprised to see such differences for the same testing, for example in Canada and the US where there is a lot of difference in these costs per QALY. So, even for the same type of testing different costs are calculated; that is what surprised me.

S.L. Stramer: For the same tests the costs are calculated differently. Well, I mean they are relatively comparable for HIV and HCV NAT.

J. Marcelis: I just understood dr. de Wolf had a test for TTV and there is relation between TTV and hepatitis B. I suppose that we introduce TTV testing, because there is a test. So, politicians will ask us to carry out this test. Is that a correct interpretation of your lecture dr. de Wolf?

J.Th.M. de Wolf: Yes, that surprised me.

C.Th. Smit Sibinga: Dr. Smit, you were absolutely clear that heterozygotes for metabolic diseases should not be deferred as donors of stem cells or bone marrow, because of the metabolism of pre-enzymes in the liver of the recipient and not reaching the actual final target organ where the disorder really comes to clinical features. Does that also relate then to the mesenchymal type of stem cells.

G.P.A. Smit: That is a different approach. The first part of my presentation was about donor suitability; that means a patient or a relative of a patient with a metabolic disease should he be accepted as a potential donor or not. I think even when a patient with phenylketonuria is used as donor for bone marrow transplantation in an oncology patient, from the metabolic point of view there is no problem. Because even when there is a pre-enzymatic accumulation of substrate, the recipient is very well capable of handling this metabolite, because he has a normal liver activity for this enzyme. That goes for a lot of metabolic diseases. That is why we divided them in bone marrow related and non bone marrow related. When it is a non bone marrow related disease there is no problem at all. The other approach is when you want to use bone marrow transplantation as a therapeutic intervention in patients with a metabolic disease. What you want to introduce in these patients is as high as possible enzyme activity. Especially in those situations where you are missing the enzyme. But the problem is that in many of these diseases especially the lysosomal storage diseases, you cannot reach the compartment you really want the enzyme activity to be restored in; that is the cerebral compartment. The problem is the blood-brain barrier. It seems that some macrophages can cross the blood-brain barrier, transform and than produce the enzyme. That is some latest information I got from a friend in Hamburg[1] and experimentally this works. So, probably stem cell transplantation with a migration of the cells. That is why I showed you the cartoons at the end and in the beginning. We hope that this will help these patients. But the experts tell that it will never be a cure, because the enzyme activity you can restore will not be available for all the cells we want it in. I think that we just have to think of new ways in helping these patients. Enzyme replacement is certainly not the way of doing this.

C.Th. Smit Sibinga: Because there is a discrepancy at this point in time practised all over the world in relation to allogeneic stem cell transplantation. If we deal with stem cells that we recover from the umbilical cord or the placenta, mothers are heavily scrutinized for all kind of metabolic disorders. If anything is traceable in the family they are not accepted. However, if we deal with other types of allogeneic donors we do not usually ask the same type of questions, even do not bother about it. I understand from your presentation that we should not worry about the possibility, even the likelihood of transmission of a metabolic disorder through stem cell transplantation; is that correct?

1. K. Ullrich, Uniklinik Hamburg-Eppendorf, D (personal communication).

G.P.A. Smit: I specifically used as an example the homozygous patient with phenylketonuria, where we might collect stem cells from heterozygotes. Of course, if you take an at random sample of umbilical cord blood and you collect stem cells, than you have a very high chance that you will have a heterozygous sample for a metabolic disease.

C.Th. Smit Sibinga: It might be sensible to revisit these criteria and discuss them in the light of your knowledge and your experience as a true metabolic disorder specialist, rather than from the hematology side.

G.P.A. Smit: From a metabolic point of view, especially with non bone marrow related metabolic diseases, I cannot find any hesitation to use these stem cells.

M.J. Postma: To come back to a remark just made by Mr. the Wit on the problem of bacterial contamination; it is a big problem, it is said. But to me it is still a bit obscure how big the problem is. When I started to work on the bacterial contamination I had in mind five cases of bacterial sepsis per year in the Netherlands. Probably I was totally wrong. I have now seen these data from the Dutch Hospital central registration about 34 cases per year in the Netherlands, where sepsis is primary diagnosed for the hospital stay. I was just interested in hearing the opinions of more experts than myself on these numbers.

Dr. Marcelis or maybe Dr. de Wolf being clinician, may have better judgements on these numbers.

R.Y. Dodd: There are two issues here in these kinds of studies. On the one hand there is sepsis that is introduced by the transfused blood and that is perhaps where you expect to have five per year. But than there is also surgical sepsis or sepsis that will occur in patients perhaps as a result of immunomodulation brought on by the leukocytes in the transfused product. So, you may be talking about two very different kinds of phenomena. I think that is the issue that perhaps need a little more exploration. Bring up the clinicians at this point.

J.H. Marcelis: I am not a clinician, but I was wondering how are these 34 cases proven? Are they all proven by blood cultures taken from the patients and are these blood cultures compared to bacteria isolated in the transfused blood product? In the Dutch situation we see a lot of cultures made from platelets resulting in coagulase negactive staphylococci (i.e. not Staphylococcus Aureus) which we all have on our skin. If clinicians take blood cultures from patients we see that 10-20% of these are positive with coagulase negative staphylococci (CNS), depending on the quality of the skills of the nurses and the doctors in the wards. If we have only one positive blood culture with a CNS it is possibly a contaminating organism from the skin of the patient. So, we always want to see at least two or three positive blood cultures with the same CNS to decide this is the causative microorganism. Because there are many different CNS you can isolate a coagulase negative staphylococcus and you isolate CNS from the patient and the blood bag which are not the same. You need at least sophisticated techniques not present in all hospitals to prove that these bacteria are the same. So, possibly in at least some of those 34 cases CNS originate from the skin of patients. The real cause of the sepsis of the patient is not revealed but was not transfusion related although (another) CNS was isolated from the blood bag. Maybe this explains why you saw 34 cases of sepsis, but a low mortality rate. Mortality rates much lower than should be expected from the results of Dr. Blajchman.[1,2] He expected about five percent of the patients will die because of the transfusion related sepsis. Infections with CNS are not so severe as infections with serious potential pathogens like Staphyloccus Aureus, or Gram negative bacteria. Do you know anything about the kind of bacteria which were detected in these 34 cases?

M. J. Postma: The kind of bacteria is not mentioned is this registration. This is a registration of individual doctors who give their figures to the central body. I would suspect that not in every case, culture is even done. We had some experience with pneumococcemia in the past and than we also saw that the pneumococcosis is not always cultured. Of course this is different, but it is all individual clinicians. The nice thing is, it is a central registration, but how the clinicians register, only the clinicians themselves know.

D. S. Wages: Yes, I can comment further on Dr. Marcelis' point. Recently, Baxter Cerus Corporation actually finished the clinical trial in Europe and in the United States for the pathogen inactivation system. As part of the trial they introduced into the protocol a system where, if a patient had a septic episode or had been cultured for any reason, the platelet unit under investigation also had to be cultured. At the end of the study it turns out to be that the positive cultures just reflected the background contamination that occurred in micro-biology laboratories in general. This happens all the time throughout any clinical laboratory in any hospital. That turned out to be a significant problem. The only way to truly resolve the issue in the Baxter-Cerus study was in fact to have a very stringent set of criteria which frankly I doubt has been employed for any of these epidemiological surveys. So, I think that is a point that when we look at these data to recognize that there are a lot of potential problems with interpreting what the true incidents of sepsis – truly due to transfusion – is. Also one should bear in mind that what we are really concerned about is clinically significant sepsis or transmission bacteria, we're all bacteriemic transiently when we brush our teeth for example. But to address this issue in the context of approach a clinical trial, our criteria were: You had to have the exact identical species present in the patient, in the blood component of interest. It has to meet the criteria for not being a background contaminate in the clinical laboratory. You have to have conclusively show that the bacteria isolated from the patient and that isolated from the container of the transfused unit were identical. That is not standard practice. That only occurred in the context of this clinical trial. I do not

---

1. Blajchman MA, Ali AM, Richardson HL. Bacterial contamination of cellular blood components. Vox Sang 1994;67(suppl):464-69.
2. Blajchman MA. Bacterial contamination and proliferation during the storage of cellular blood products. Vox Sang 1998;74(suppl 2):155-59.

think that that would be feasible in an epidemiological manner throughout the country.

D. S. Wages: That is very true. My recollection is that one of the good things about the hemovigilance system in France is that in each case an attempt was made to characterize each report on a four point scale from meaningless to almost certainly confirmed. There was a very large number of cases that went into the tunnel and a very small number of cases that were actually confirmed to be transfusion associated sepsis. So, perhaps you're seeing the broader end of the funnel also.

J.H. Marcelis: You are correct. I don't know the numbers exactly, but they started with forty-three and I thought they ended seven proven cases, something like that. If you do this kind of testing, you still must be very careful because we also run a transfusion laboratory in a hospital. The moment a patient develops a fever period during transfusion the nurse runs to the patient, pulls everything out, puts it in a big bag, sends it back to the laboratory and screams: "Transfusion reaction". Than you get some bloody giving set and you have to take out blood and it's almost unavoidable that you have the same bacteria in this blood bag, which obviously came from the patient. Professor Claes Högman[1] told me that he had positive blood cultures of a patient and there were also positive cultures from a blood product and it was a Gram negative bacterium. They thought that was an infection due to the transfusion. However, when they looked better, they saw that the patient had already positive blood cultures that were taken twelve hours before. So the patient inocculated the blood product, so I think if we start hemovigilance on this we must also have very good instructions to our nurses, to the clinicians, to have a real good hemovigilance system. Of course, actually one central laboratory which could pick up all the strains by sophisticated molecular biology technology would be appropriate.

D. S. Wages: I just want to follow up to that. I think that is valuable in theory. I would find it very hard to believe that in a real hospital without people concerned about a particular trial, that you could do this for all transfusions throughout the year. I just doubt that that is logistically feasible.

J.H. Marcelis: I'm afraid of that too. But at least you could ask them to put a cover on the needle and then bring it back properly.

B. Ekermo (Linköping, S): I have two comments. First, an earlier speaker said that the regulators, when they introduce new tests, find it difficult to withdraw them. In Sweden we have an example from seven years ago; there was a regulation that we had to test every donation for anti-HTLV I and II. After one year testing they evaluated the results and now we are only testing every donor once. So, that gives hope for regulations in Sweden.

1. Högman CF. A brief review of bacterial contamination of blood components. Vox Sang 1996;70(suppl 3):78-82.

Another comment related to NA-Testing of donors. In Sweden there has been documented outbreaks of Hepatitis C in a haematology ward [1] and in pediatric oncology service. One of the authors has put forward the provoking question: In a system with limited health care resources, like in Sweden where we have mainly public health care, if you divert money and resources to NAT of blood donors, will this increase the total spread of nosocomial infections? Because, you can hire less nurses, they get a more stressful working situation and they may make more mistakes with needles and so. In one of these outbreaks the main reason for the spread of hepatitis C was thought to be the use of multidose vials for dugs and i.v. solutions. When the stressed nurse wanted to pick up more drug or i.v. solution from the multidose vial, she forgot to change to a clean syringe and inoculated the multidose vial with blood from the patient who might have been hepatitis C positive. After that every new patient receiving drug/i.v. solution from that multidose vial got infected. A wild guess is that in Sweden perhaps there might be 200 cases of hepatitis C nosocomial transmissions in the hospitals each year and at most only one of these due to a blood component from a window phase donation. So that is what the provoking question was.

S.L. Stramer: You know, you keep adding money and by the end of the day we have to pay for the unit. We are going to have decreased services in the hospital in general and something is going to loose. Because we have to spend all this money for blood, we are not going to have money for staff. We have to fire nurses, we have to decrease staff, more errors will be made. We don't know any quantitative estimates for this yet. But that seems like a very logical scenario because there is only so much money to go around.

C.Th. Smit Sibinga: Dr. Stramer, you showed somewhere in the course of your presentation the genome HCV phenotype study. I noticed that you had a genotype 1, 2 and 6 and the 4 and 5 were missing. Was that on purpose or was that just because you did not have access?

S.L. Stramer: No, it's just what we happened to have found in our study. I mean, we had genotype 3, 1A, 1B and we didn't find any 4 and 5, just because they are rarer in the US. So is 6, and we just didn't happen to encounter those. The test has the ability to detect all genotypes, at least from the data, the manufacturers show us. They detect all genotypes, but it is just by chance, we have not found one yet because those are rare in the US.

1. Widell A, Christensson B, Wiebe T, et al. Epidemiological and molecular investigation of outbreaks of hepatitis C virus infection on a pediatric oncology service. Ann Intern Med 1999;130:130-34.

IV. PREVENTATIVE ASPECTS

QUANTITATIVE REAL-TIME PCR FOR DETECTION OF PARVOVIRUS B19 DNA IN BLOOD PLASMA FOR PLASMA SCREENING.

M.H.G.M. Koppelman, H.T.M. Cuypers[1]

Introduction

Human Parvovirus B19 (PV-B19) is a 18-26 nm small, non-enveloped, single stranded DNA virus belonging to the family Parvoviridae. The virus has a tropism for red blood cell progenitors. Most of the clinical manifestations due to viral infection are related to impairment of the functions of red blood cell progenitors (i.e. transient aplastic crisis, pure red cell aplasia) or to circulating immune complexes resulting from infection (Erythema infectiosum, rash, arthropathy). PV-B19 is normally transmitted via the respiratory route. PV-B19 is commonly found in blood donors. The prevalence of high viremic PV-B19 infection among blood donors is estimated between 1:20,000 to 1:50,000 [1]. However, during micro epidemic periods the prevalence can be as high as 1:260 [1]. The high viremic period after infection is usually short and very intense with PV-B19 loads up to 10^{14} copies /ml in plasma. After this initial burst of virus, infected individuals stay low viremic for a prolonged period up to several months with load $<10^4$ copies/ml in plasma. Although normally transmitted via the respiratory route, parental transmission of PV-B19 can occur via the administration of blood components and blood derivatives. Transmission via blood components originating from a single donor occurs only rarely. The reported cases include a recipient of an infected red cell unit with thalassemia [2] and recipients who underwent bone marrow [3] or liver transplantation. These rare observations are in contrast with many reports on the transmission of PV-B19 via blood derivatives such as clotting factor concentrates, albumin and IVIG [4].

A substantial part (40-60 %) of the large pools of plasma (usually > 5000 donations per pool) for production of blood derivatives contain measurable PV-B19 DNA by PCR, due to the prevalence of infection and the fact that PV-B19 infected individuals stay low viremic in the plasma for quite a long period after the first burst of virus. However, only one third of these production pools are high viremic as result of contamination with a high load plasma unit [5]. Solvent detergent or heat treatment can not always prevent PV-B19 transmission by blood derivatives due to the non-enveloped and heat resistant nature of PV-B19. As outcome of the VITEX study [1] it became clear, that removal of high load PV-B19 units leads to manufacturing pools of plasma with a load below 10^4 copies/ml. Solvent detergent treated plasma produced from these pools with a

1. Sanquin Diagnostics Viral Serology, Amsterdam, NL.

load < 10^4 copies/ml proved be save for PV-B19 transmission. When manufacturers want to improve the safety of the blood derivatives with regard to PV-B19, manufacturing pools should be prepared with PV-B19 levels below 10^4 copies/ml (FDA's perspective [1]). To accomplish this objective, high load units should be removed by means of screening of test pools prepared from the test tubes representative for the plasma units. Test pools composed of 100-500 units are used by several manufacturer's and blood transfusion organizations. These test pools have to be analyzed with a quantitative test for PV-B19 DNA. When the PV-B19 load is above the limit for acceptation of the test pool, smaller pools are composed, in order to track down the unit(s) responsible for the high load in the test pool. The limits for acceptation and rejection are presented in Table 1. The system contains an additional safety factor of 10 between test pool and production pool, in order to be sure that the guideline of lower than 10^4 copies/ml PV-B19 DNA can be reached.

Table 1: PV-B19 DNA limits for release or rejection of plasma and plasma pools

Plasma	Limit (IU/mL)
Individual donation	5×10^6
Test pool of 8 donations	6×10^5
Test pool of 48 donations	10^5
Test pool of 480 donations	10^4
Manufacturing pool	10^4

We have evaluated the use of real time PCR for quantitative detection of PV-B19 DNA.for the screening of manufacturing plasma by means of test pools. The real-time PCR was performed on the LightCycler [6]. This instrument makes it possible to perform a PCR reaction and to follow the formation of the product during the amplification reaction by means of hybridization with fluorophore-labeled probes. The experimental test for quantitative detection of PV-B19 DNA used in this evaluation was developed by Roche Diagnostics. The test was performed in combination with extraction with silica particles of pooled plasma (Boom technology [7]), using the NucliSens extractor (bioMérieux). We evaluated the analytical aspects; linearity, and precision. The conversion factor between copies determined in this test and International Units (IU) as defined on the International Standard Parvovirus B19 DNA from WHO [8] was determined. Hundred samples from manufacturing pools and 50 from test pools of 480 donations have been analyzed to determine the utility of the test in plasma screening.

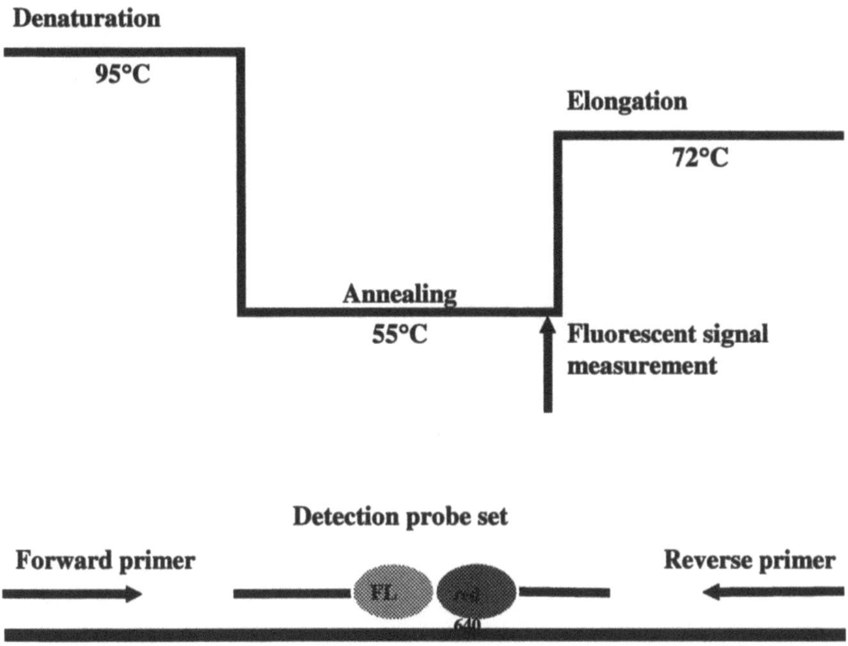

Figure 1. Figure 1: Principle of PV-B19 DNA LightCycler test. Both primers and detection probes hybridize to target DNA during the annealing phase of PCR. The fluorophores of the detection probes come in close proximity. Fluorescein (FL) is exited by the LightCycler. Part of the excitation energy will be transferred to LC-Red-640. LC-Red-640 will emit light that is measured.

Quantitative real-time PCR detection of Parvo B19 DNA on the LightCycler

The principle of real-time PCR is depicted in Figure 1. After nucleic acid extraction, target PV-B19 sequences are amplified with specific primers in the PCR reaction in incubation capillaries. These capillaries can be irradiated in the LightCycler with a laser during programmed periods and at the same time emitted light is measured with a photo-multiplier tube. Specific detection with hybridization probes of amplification product is achieved during the annealing phase of each PCR cycle. Hybridization probes are a pair of oligo-nucleotides labeled with two different fluorophores. One oligo is labeled at the 3'-end with fluorescein, which serves as the donor fluorophore. The other oligo is labeled 5'-end with LightCycler red 640 (acceptor fluorophore). Upon binding of the hybridization probes to PV-B19 amplification product both donor and acceptor fluorophores come in close proximity, resulting in Fluorescence Resonance Energy Transfer (FRET) between both fluorophores. Fluorescein is excited by the LightCycler laser (470nm) and part of the excitation energy is transferred to the acceptor fluorophore. The acceptor fluorophore starts to emit fluorescent signal at 640 nm. The fluorescent signal is measured by the photo-multiplier

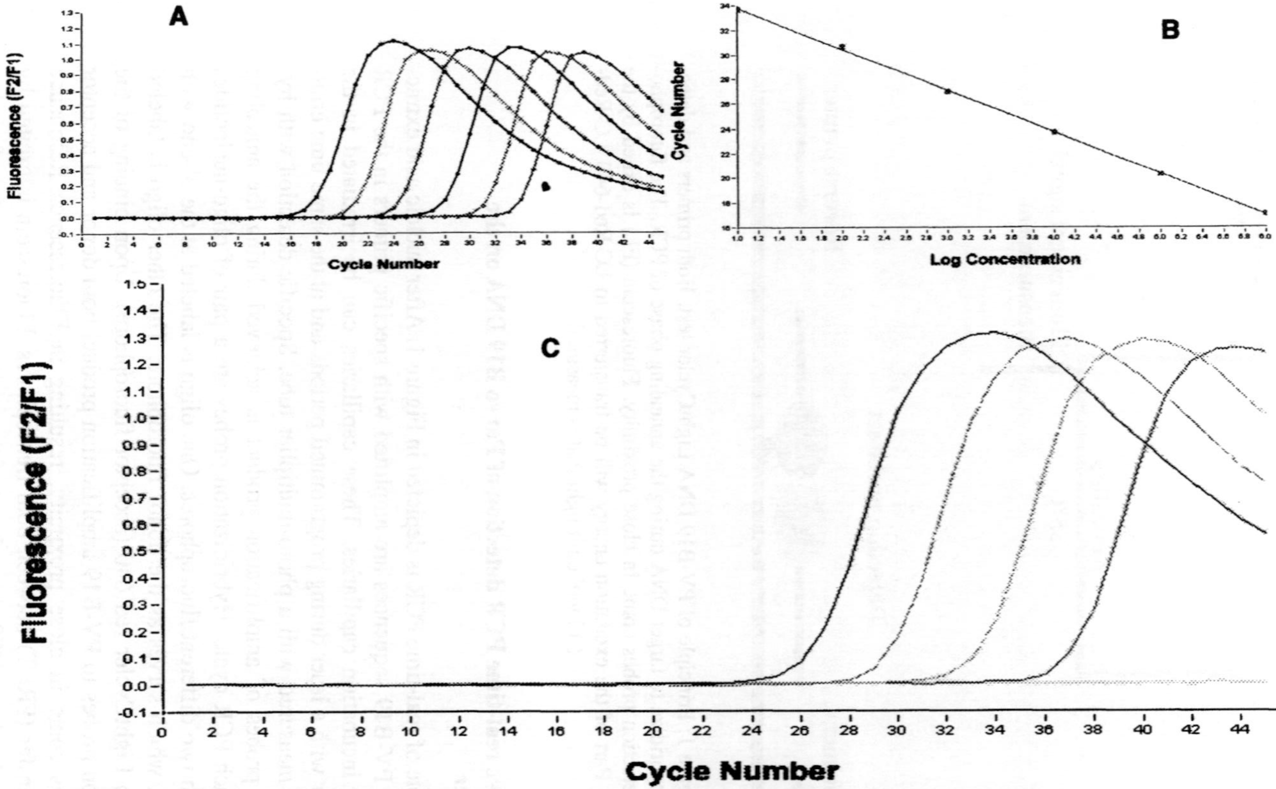

Figure 2. Typical results of the PV-B19 LightCycler test. Amplification of calibration standards. From left to right 10^6, 10^5, 10^4, 10^3, 10^2, 10^1 PV B19-DNA copies/capillary. Calibration curve based on the Crossing Points (CP) and the input concentrations of calibration standards. Ten-fold dilution series of IS B19-DNA. From left to right 10^5, 10^4, 10^3, 10^2 and 10 IU/mL.

tube. The emitted signal is a measure for the amount of generated PCR product. To quantify the PV-B19 DNA load in the nucleic acid extract, PV-B19 DNA external standards with a known B19 DNA copy number are included in the test. A typical real-time PCR result of external standards is shown in Figure 2A. Six standards with respectively 10^6, 10^5, 10^4, 10^3, 10^2 and 10^1 Parvo B19 DNA copies/test capillary were amplified in the presence of PV-B19 specific hybridization probes. From the log-linear phase of each of the standards the so-called crossing point on the x-axis is calculated based on the second derivative method and expressed as cycle number. The crossing points are used to draw the calibration curve, Figure 2B. The quantity of PV-B19 DNA in test samples is read out from the calibration curve. Results of WHO IS PV-B19 reference material in a 10-fold dilution series are depicted in Figure 2C.

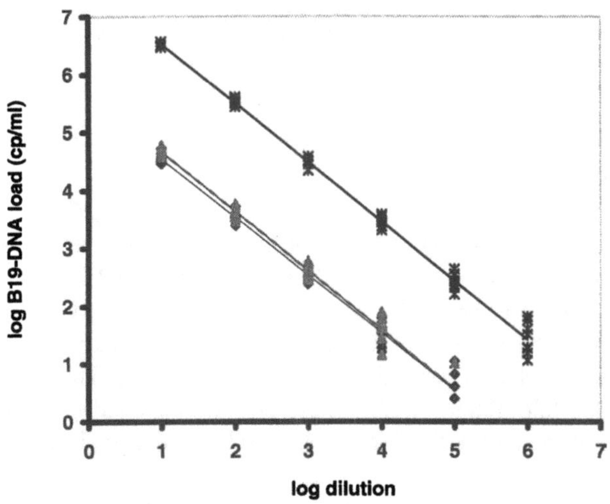

Figure 3. PV-B19 DNA load in dilution series of IS PV-B19 DNA (◆), PV-B19 reference sample CC (▲) and PV B19 reference sample DD (✳). Eight replicas of each dilution were tested. Test results are depicted log transformed and plotted against the

log dilution.

Analytical Validation of the LightCycler Parvovirus B19 quantitative test

PV-B19 DNA content was determined in dilution series of the WHO International Standard for PV-B19 DNA (IS PV-B19 DNA: 10^6 IU/ml) and in dilution series of two other reference materials; CC (CBER/FDA, Rockville, USA) and DD (VQC-CLB, Amsterdam, The Netherlands). These three reference materials were already evaluated in the collaborative study to characterize the IS PV-B19 [8]. Data from the collaborative study are compared with results of the PV-B19 LightCycler test. Ten fold dilution series of each reference material were analyzed in eight fold in the PV-B19 LightCycler test. To analyze linearity and precision, results were log transformed and plotted against the log dilution (Figure 3). In the range 10^3-10^5 IU/ml a high precision was found (Table 2) with standard deviation values of 0.08-0.13 log. At lower PV-B19 DNA content the

Table 2: Precision (=standard deviation) and accuracy (difference between input and output load) of the PV-B19 LightCycler test. Eight replicas of each member of IS PV B19-DNA dilution series were tested. The output PV-B19 DNA load is presented in IU/mL

Input (IU/mL)	log Input (IU/mL)	N*	N-pos**	N-neg***	log Output (IU/mL)****	Precision	Accuracy
10	1.00	8	4	4	1.17	0.28	0.17
100	2.00	8	8	0	1.91	0.19	0.09
1,000	3.00	8	8	0	2.99	0.13	0.01
10,000	4.00	8	8	0	4.00	0.10	0.00
100,000	5.00	8	8	0	4.99	0.08	0.01

* N= number of samples tested.
** N-pos =number of positive results
*** N-neg = number of negative results
**** Conversion factor copies to IU=2.84

precision decreased to 0.28 log at 10 IU/ml. At the limit for release or rejection of plasma for manufacturing (10^4 IU/ml) the mean measured value was exactly 10,000 IU/ml with lower and upper limit of 8,240 and 12,200 IU/ml (95 % confidence interval). The potency of standard CC and DD relative to IS PV-B19 DNA was determined with parallel line analysis (Figure 3). The replicas of the 10-fold and 1000-fold dilution were used to perform the analysis because of the high precision of the test in this range. The results of this analyses are summarized in Table 3. The potencies of standard CC and DD relative to AA as determined with the LightCycler test and the values obtained in the WHO study were comparable. Values of the 95 % confidence interval for the potencies in the LightCycler test reveal that the real time PCR test is very precise. The maximum and minimum values for the potencies in the collaborative WHO study based on the maximum likelihood method showed a much higher variation, probably as result of the heterogeneity of used extraction and amplification methods. The conversion factor from copies in the LightCycler test to IU defined on IS PV-B19 DNA was determined on the results of the dilution series of the interna tional standard (Figure 4). The conversion factor was calculated as 2.84 from the Y-intercept (95% confidence interval 1.71 - 4.72).

Parvo B19 in plasma pools

PV-B19 was determined in manufacturing pools (approximately 5000 donations) and in test pools of 480 donations. Nucleic acid extract was prepared from 1 ml of pooled plasma with the NucliSens extractor and analyzed for PV B19 DNA content with the LightCycler test. Retrospectively a total of 100 manufaturing pools of Sanquin Plasmaproducts representative for the year 2000 was analyzed (Figure 5). Six pools had a Parvo B19 load of >10^4 IU/ml and should

Table 3: Calibration of PV-B19 DNA reference samples (CC and DD). Comparison between PV B19 LightCycler test and results from the WHO collaborative study [8]. Standards CC and DD were provided by CBER/FDA and VQC-Sanquin respectively

Reference Sample	PV B19 LightCycler test		WHO collaborative study	
	Potency	**95%CI***	**Mean Potency**	**Min – Max****
CC	1.21	1.06 – 1.38	1.15	0.03 – 89.13
DD	88.04	71.52 – 108.39	89.13	7.59 – 2344

* 95% CI= 95% confidence interval.
** Min – Max = lowest and highest potency found in the WHO collaborative study.

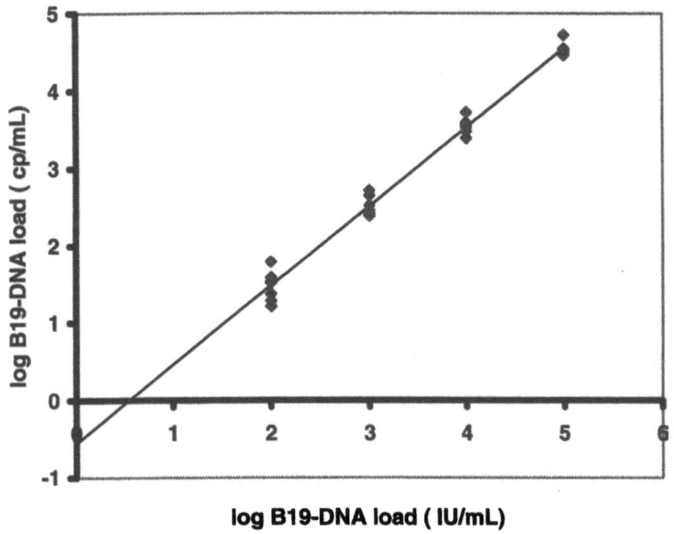

Figure 4: Determination of the conversion factor from copies to International Units for the PV B19 LightCycler test. Eight replicas of each member of IS PV-B19 DNA dilution series were tested. Test results are depicted log transformed and plotted against the log input (IU/mL).

have been rejected for production of plasma products, when the guideline for the reduction of the PV-B19 content would have been in practice. The observed data are comparable with the results published by another manufacturer (Gross et al.: presentation ISBT July 2000, Vienna).

The prevalence of blood donors highly viremic for PV-B19 was determined with test pools (480 donations) during the first half of 2001 under 24,000 randomly selected blood donors. Results are depicted in Table 4 for late winter/start of spring (March April) and for spring/start summer (May-July). Test pools with

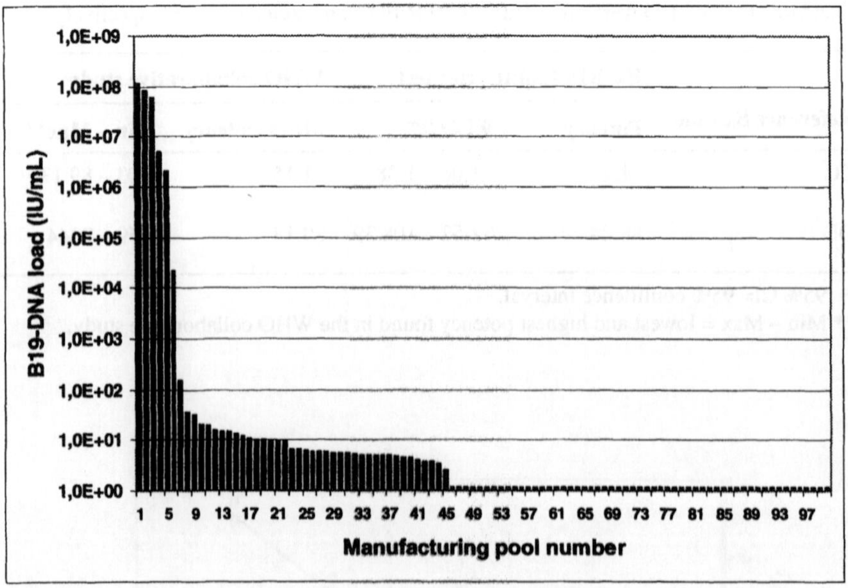

Figure 5: PV-B19 DNA load in 100 manufacturing pools representative for year 2000 (Sanquin Plasmaproducts).

Table 4: PV-B19 DNA load in test pools of 480 donations. Test pools were prepared from donations collected in two different periods in 2001

Period in 2001	Number of $pools^{480}$ tested	Number of test pools of 480 donations with PV-B19 DNA load (IU/mL) in indicated range				
		0	$1\text{-}10^2$	$10^2\text{-}10^4$	$10^4\text{-}10^7$	$>10^7$
March/April	20	4	1	8	0	7
May/June/July	30	19	1	10	0	0
Total	50	23	2	18	0	7

a high PV-B19 DNA load (> 10^7 IU/ml) were only found during the first period, although more donors were tested during the second period. Brake down of the test pools to the individual high viremic donations by means of testing test pools of 48, and 8 donations revealed a number of 7 high viremic donations. Based on these data a prevalence of high viremic donations was calculated of 1 in 3,500 for this period. A comparable survey testing 30,000 donors in April - June 2002 revealed a prevalence for high viremic donations of 1 in 10,000 (results not further shown).

Final remarks

Preceded by HIV-RNA, HCV RNA, and HBV DNA, PV-B19-DNA is the next target for nucleic acid amplification technology (NAT) to further improve the safety of blood derivatives with respect to viral transmission. PV-B19 infection is probably quite harmless for healthy individuals. In contrast, special groups of patients like individuals with high red cell turnover due to hemolysis, blood loss and so forth, PV-B19 infection can lead to an "aplastic crisis". Pregnant women in the second trimester and immunosuppressed patients (i.e. congenital immunodeficiency, AIDS, lymphoproliferative disorders and transplantation patients) also represent a group at risk. Under these risk groups some patients are frequent users of blood derivatives as result of therapeutic intervention. In the approach to improve continuously the safety with regard to viral infections for recipients of blood derivatives, the European Pharmacopea has planned to add prescreening of pooled plasma for the manufacturing of anti-D immunoglobulin to the monograph for plasma in January 2003. This approach to protect pregnant women with a higher risk of adverse effects for the child in case of PV-B19 infection is realized by limiting the potential PV-B19 virus burden in the manufacturing pools by testing with a quantitative PV-B19 NAT assay and excluding the pools with a load > 10^4 IU/ml. To prevent large losses of plasma it is necessary to pre-screen the plasma and to remove the high load PV-B19 units. This approach presumes the use of a quantitative PV-B19 DNA assay, which is precise in the range 10^3-10^5 IU/ml. The results with the experimental PV-B19 LightCycler test reveal a high precision over this range of less then 0.13 log. Positive controls at the level of 10^4 IU/ml for release or rejection of manufacturing pools as prescribed in the Pharmacopea, are quantified in 96% of the assays in the range between 6300 IU/ml 15900 IU/ml (mean ± 2 SD). Results of calculated potencies between reference material obtained with the PV-B19 LightCycler test and the results obtained in the collaborative study of WHO are comparable. The WHO results are compiled from a number of different NAT tests. This comparison indicates, that secondary reference materials can be calibrated against the international standard in a reproducible manner. The determination of the conversion factor between copies based on the calibration standards of LightCycler test and international units (IU) makes it possible to express the results of the real time PCR test in IU. It is obvious, based on a representative analyses of manufacturing pools of the year 2000, that a substantial loss of production plasma will take place in case of exclusion of pools with a B19 DNA load greater than 10^4 IU/ml, when no pre-screening of plasma units is implemented. The small pilot screening in spring 2001 indicated, that the prevalence will change with the season. The consequence of this is a large difference in workload for the screenings laboratory performing the analyses for PV-B19 DNA for plasma release purposes, depending on the seasonal period.

In this study a prototype version of the quantitative PV-B19 LightCycler test was evaluated. Based on the encouraging results with this experimental assay Roche Diagnostics developed a commercial version of the LightCycler test. The commercial test includes the use of internal control molecules, which make it possible to control the extraction and amplification procedure to prevent "false negative" results due to inadequate extraction or inhibition of amplification by disturbing substances. The internal control (IC) molecules are amplified with the same oligo-nucleotide for amplification. Within the amplified region, a nucleotide sequence is mutated, to make detection of IC-amplicons possible with a IC-specific pair of hybridization probes. The IC-specific hybridization probes are labeled with an acceptor fluorophores, which excites light at another wavelength than for the wild-type target (705 nm instead of 640 nm). This test is now under evaluation.

Acknowledgements

The authors want to thank Dr. Thomas Emrich of Roche Diagnostics RandD facilities (Penzberg, Germany) for making available the experimental PV-B19 DNA test and for stimulating cooperation during this evaluation.

References

1. Brown KE, Young NS, Alving BM, Barbosa LH. Parvovirus B19: implications for transfusion medicine. Summary of a workshop. Transfusion 2001; 41:130-35.
2. Zanella A, Rossi F, Cesana C, et al. Transfusion-transmitted human parvovirus B19 infection in a thalassemic patient. Transfusion 1995;35:769-72.
3. Cohen BJ, Beard S, Knowles WA, et al. Chronic anemia due to parvovirus B19 infection in a bone marrow transplant patient after platelet transfusion. Transfusion 1997;37:947-52.
4. Azzi A, Morfini M, Mannucci PM. The transfusion-associated transmission of parvovirus B19. Transfus Med Rev 1999;13:194-204.
5. Schmidt I, Blumel J, Seitz H, Willkommen H, Lower J. Parvovirus B19 DNA in plasma pools and plasma derivatives. Vox Sang. 2001;81:228-35.
6. Wittwer CT, Ririe KM, Andrew RV, David DA, Gundry RA, Balis UJ. The LightCycler: a microvolume multisample fluorimeter with rapid temperature control. Biotechniques 1997;22:176-81.
7. Boom R, Sol CJ, Salimans MM, et al. Rapid and simple method for purification of nucleic acids. J Clin Microbiol 1990;28:495-503.
8. Saldanha J, Lelie N, Yu MW, Heath A. Establishment of the first World Health Organization International Standard for human parvovirus B19 DNA nucleic acid amplification techniques. Vox Sang 202;82:24-31.

ADVANCES IN BACTERIAL DETECTION TECHNOLOGY

Willem P.A. van der Tuuk Adriani[1] and Cees Th. Smit Sibinga[2]

Introduction

A few decades ago bacteriology was an important item in the entire cycle of blood transfusion; from collecting whole blood to administration of blood products. All attempts to solve the problems turning up in the field of virology, bacteriology was more and more pushed to the background.
Prior to pay attention to new advanced technology in detection of microbials it is necessary to fresh up our memory.

The first question that rises is: what kind of products are our blood products in terms of legislation. Of course blood products are transplants, but there is no law concerning this kind of products. On the other hand it is clear that blood products are no common ware like toys. In our point of view they are medicinal products. To prove this statement we have translated the definition of a medicinal product as it is defined the Dutch Drug Act (art. 1) [1].
A medicinal product is a substance or a composition of substances that is used or recommended to be suitable to:

- cure, relieve or prevent any illness, disease, or wound in humans;
- to improve or repair the function of human organs;
- diagnose by application to humans.

If we change the word 'substance' in 'tissue' we have an good and practical definition. This definition, however, does not say anything about the route of administration and its consequences.

Blood products are parenteral administered and therefore must be sterile [2]. As a consequence blood products must be processed under aseptic conditions where sterilization is impossible. Now we have to ask ourselves two important questions:

- Are blood products indeed sterile?
- What does sterile actually means?

---

1. Manager Quality Assurance, Sanquin Division Blood Bank Noord Nederland, Groningen, NL.
2. Director WHO Collaborating Center for Blood Transfusion and Sanquin Consulting Services, Blood Bank Noord Nederland, Groningen, NL.Vice-president, AABB Consulting Services Division, Groningen, NL.

Sterility and blood products

Sterility is an absolute term and it is difficult to prove that a product is sterile [3]. If we take an aliquot of a batch that is sterilized and no micro-organism is found it does not guarantee that the entire batch does not contain any micro-organisms. To solve this problem the international pharmaceutical industry has agreed that a product may be claimed to be sterile if the risk of contamination is less than one to a million ($< 1 \times 10^6$). The validation of the sterilization process is the basis for the prove of batch sterility. How to do this?

Produce a batch of the product that needs to be sterile under the described normal standard conditions. Contaminate this finished batch with a known – quantitatively and qualitatively – micro-organism. Mix well and determine the starting contamination level. Start now the sterilization process and take samples in the course of the time or irradiation level – depending on the sterilization method. Determine the contamination level of each sample and plot the results on semi-logarithmic paper. A straight line will appear as shown below. The line may of course be extrapolated when the zero level is reached till the end of the sterilization process. From this plot the number of log-units from start to finish can be easily read. This is the so called D-value. This D-value must be larger than 6. In the example given below the D-value is 8. This means that the maximum starting level of contamination of the batches of this product produced in the future must be 100 (= 10^2). The validation of the sterilization process has proved that with a starting level of $< 10^2$ the end level will be $< 10^{-6}$.
Back to our precious blood products it will now be clear that blood products can by definition not be claimed to be sterile. As a consequence the aseptic conditions during the entire processing of blood and blood products is of critical importance. This process starts with the donor selection. Observe the skin of the donor as much as possible to see whether there are infectious wounds and ask the donor for treatment by a dentist during the last three day prior to donation.

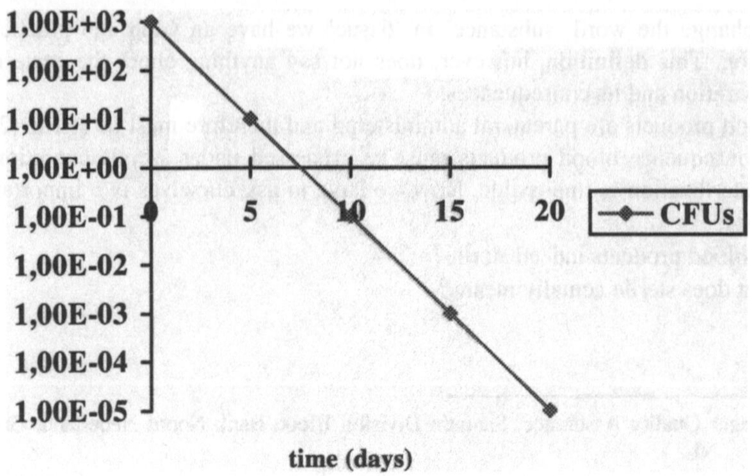

D-value determination

The second critical point is the venepuncture. Disinfection of the venepuncture site, the finger tips of the phlebotomist in case of palpation and the puncture technique are important. If the needle is inserted straight a part of the skin will be changed in a kind of valve; if the needle is rotated during the puncture a part of the skin will be drilled out and will be part of the first volume of blood collected. Since the further processing is performed in closed blood bag systems normal hygiene and GMP conditions are sufficient to exclude the risk of contamination.

The above stated importance of the aseptic conditions require a good monitoring of the process. The most risky product that is produced by each blood bank is the platelet concentrate. The process is the most complicated (connection of several bags to pool a number of buffy coats) and the storage conditions (room temperature) are favorable for bacteria to grow. Therefore platelet concentrates are the products of concern for a good monitoring process. By Dutch law all platelet concentrates must be checked for bacterial growth since November first, 2001.

Experience

The Blood Bank Noord Nederland has over two years experience monitoring 100% of all platelets concentrates. Every finished product is sampled under aseptic conditions using a laminar flow hood. The samples are cultured in the BacT/Alert® (Organon Teknika). During the first 24 hours after preparation the products are in principle not distributed to the hospitals. Thereafter they are issued negative to date.

As the rate of positive culture results is low the following assumption is justified: If we find a positive result on a sample of PC 5U, this contamination is due to only one of the constituting donations. This leads to the following calculation:

Number of samples from the various products + (3 times the number of samples from PC 3U) + (5 times the number of samples from PC 5U) gives the number of donations that are tested for bacterial contamination.

Using this monitoring system and calculation method we got the following results: 35,000 donations were tested out of 80.000 whole blood donations: 0.1 - 0.2% is contaminated.

Available technology

Until recent classical culture techniques were available. The most common technique is the agar plate method. This method is reliable, uses small size samples and gives the results within 3 – 4 days.

At present the BacT/Alert is the standard technique in the blood bank and many other micro-biological laboratories. It is an automated system, using a large sample volume (5-10 mL). It is quite sensitive 10^{-6} 100 CFUs/mL, but it takes 7 days to be sure to have a negative culture result.

A few new techniques are under development: Non amplified probe directed at bacterial 4.5S RNA uses a solid phase capture gel and electrophoresis followed by chemiluminescent probe; detection sensitivity 10^3 CFU/mL. This method is tested for the following micro-organisms:

- Bacillus cereus;
- Escherichia coli;
- Enterobacter Cloacae;
- Klebsiella pneumoniae;
- Pseudomonas aeruginosa;
- Serratia marcescens;
- Staphylococcus aureus, epidermidis etc..

The second new method is:
Microvolume Fluorimetry using antibiotic-labeled probes combined with microvolume fluorimetry

- sensitivity 10^3 CFU/mL;
- results within 30-40 minutes.

References

1. Dutch Drug Act. Vermande Publ. The Hague, 1997.
2. Pharmacopoeia Eur. SDU Publ. The Hague, 2001.
3. Guideline Sterilization and Sterility. Bohn, Stafleu, van Loghem Publ. Houten, 2001.

PATHOGEN INACTIVATED BLOOD COMPONENTS: ADVANCING FROM THEORY TO PRACTICE

M. Conlan, L. Corash, D. Ramies, David S. Wages[1]

Introduction

Although the safety of the blood supply has been dramatically improved over the past two decades, allogeneic blood components still carry infectious risks. This is in marked contrast to other therapeutic compounds such as small molecules or even recombinant biologics such as insulin or growth factors. Currently, prevention of transfusion-associated disease depends on a pre-donation interview of potential donors followed by laboratory testing of the donor's blood for infectious pathogens prior to release of the donor's blood. Serologic testing is performed to detect retroviruses such as the Human Immunodeficiency Virus (HIV) as well as a number of the hepatitis viruses such as hepatitis B. Serologic screening is not routinely done for parvo virus B19, hepatitis A, E and G. Further, with one exception, no screening tests for bacteria or protozoa exist. Recently, the scope and sensitivity of donor screening for viral infection has expanded by the addition of specific nucleic acid amplification tests. The addition of these screening tests has greatly narrowed the "window period" in which a seronegative donor might still transmit a viral infection.

Despite these continued improvements in pre-transfusion donor screening and testing to detect viruses associated with transfusion-transmitted infections, blood components continue to carry the risk of infectious disease [1]. Even with the introduction of nucleic acid amplification testing, there are still reports of transfusion-associated HIV or hepatitis C [2,3]. Transfusion-transmitted sepsis continues to be an ever-present risk [4].

All of the screening tests rely on an understanding of the identity of the infectious organisms that can contaminate blood. In addition, except for the test for syphilis, all of these screening tests are for viral infection. There are no prospective screening tests for bacterial contamination of a blood component. This is important, because the very success of viral screening has made the likelihood of bacterial infection much greater than the risk of viral infection [5]. Further, where there is no test for the relevant agent, such as malaria or prions, medical history based on travel and potential exposure is used to eliminate donors who could potentially transmit an infectious agent. Yet the use of an interview as opposed to a specific laboratory test greatly reduces the efficiency of screening.

---

1. Medical Affairs, Cerus Corporation 2525 Stanwell Drive, Concord, CA 94520 david_wages@ceruscorp.com The author has equity in Cerus Corporation.

This has the result of reducing the number of potential donors when the blood supply is already plagued with periodic shortages. In addition to the effect that screening procedures have on blood donations, there has been increased concern about the additional cost the vast panoply of screening tests brings to transfusion medicine [6].

Despite these problems, it should be emphasized that the approach to enhancing safety by donor screening methods works. The blood supply is safer than it has ever been. Nonetheless, there are obvious deficiencies with the current approach, which do not lend themselves to cost-effective donor screening. The point of diminishing returns has clearly been reached for screening techniques for existing viruses with no method in place to deal with the inevitable new virus when it enters the blood supply. In addition, donors are not screened for exotic agents such as protozoa, yet these represent a real threat due to increased travel and immigration.

There is thus a need for a complementary approach to maintaining blood safety. A system of inactivating pathogens present in donated blood represents a very attractive supplement to preventive screening measures. While screening techniques are very specific, any pathogen inactivation process must have broad capabilities to deal with the wide spectrum of potentially infectious pathogens. In addition, a technology that can inactivate leukocytes as well as pathogens offers important corollary benefits. Residual donor leukocytes can be associated with a spectrum of adverse events, ranging from relatively benign effects such as febrile non-hemolytic transfusion reactions to fatal transfusion-associated Graft-versus-Host Disease.

Effective pathogen inactivation is important for several reasons.

- Pathogen inactivation is an important step forward towards the goal of an almost risk-free blood supply.
- Pathogen inactivation is a breakthrough in transfusion medicine because it has the potential to inactivate pathogens that medical science has yet to identify, and more than we test for today.
- Pathogen inactivation technology is a prospective step that blood centers and hospitals can take to enhance the safety of blood transfusions.

One approach to inactivation of pathogens is to target the nucleic acid of pathogens present in prepared blood components. While all known pathogens, with the possible exception of prions, are dependent on nucleic acid for replication, no blood component requires nucleic acid for its therapeutic efficacy. Targeting nucleic acids thus represents a promising approach to pathogen inactivation. Cerus Corporation, a partner with Baxter Healthcare, has developed Helinx™ technology, which uses this approach, and Baxter Healthcare's Intercept Blood Systems are based on Helinx™ technology. This approach does not address the (currently theoretical) risk of prions, but it offers the added advantage of preventing deleterious effects from passenger leukocytes which are present in platelets and plasma even after leukocyte reduction.

This article focuses on the clinical trials of blood components prepared with Helinx™ technology. Development of effective pathogen inactivation systems must take into account the properties of different blood components. For platelets and plasma, Baxter Healthcare and Cerus Corporation have developed a photochemical treatment system using the psoralen amotosalen hydrochloride (HCl) (S-59) and ultraviolet A light. Recently, investigators participating in multi-center trials have completed pivotal trials evaluating the clinical efficacy of pathogen inactivated platelets and plasma.

A separate system has also been developed for pathogen inactivation of red blood cell (RBC) concentrates. The approach to pathogen inactivation of RBCs does not employ a photochemical treatment because the viscosity and hemoglobin concentration in RBCs prohibit use of illumination. Instead of using a psoralen, successful pathogen inactivation has been achieved using a non-light sensitive nucleic acid-targeted compound designated S-303. Initial Phase I studies of this RBC system have been completed, and pivotal trials to examine the efficacy of S-303 treated RBCs will soon begin.

Clinical trials of platelets and plasma

The novel psoralen amotosalen HCl (commonly referred to as S-59) is a planar positively charged molecule that intercalates into the double stranded regions of both DNA and RNA. When illuminated with the appropriate frequency of long wave ultraviolet light (UVA), S-59 can form a mono-adduct by co-valently attaching to one of the strands of nucleic acid. Reaction with an additional photon can cause the mono-adduct to react with the opposite nucleic acid strand and produce an inter-strand cross-link. An extensive series of experiments have shown that platelets and plasma deliberately "spiked" with high titers of viruses and bacteria are effectively treated with S-59 photochemical treatment [7]. This work has been convincingly supplemented by a chimpanzee infection study. Lin and co-workers demonstrated that full-sized human platelet concentrates (approximately 300 mL) contaminated with high titers of hepatitis B and C virus did not result in infection after transfusion into healthy chimpanzees [8]. In addition to pathogen inactivation studies, extensive nucleic acid modification by the photochemical process using S-59 shows great promise in ameliorating the detrimental effects caused by contaminating leukocytes. Platelet concentrates treated with S-59 photochemical treatment do not generate cytokines—thought to be a key factor of febrile non-hemolytic transfusion reactions. Of potentially greater significance, treatment of lymphocytes with the S-59 process prevented transfusion-associated Graft-versus-Host Disease in both healthy and immune-compromised mice in a murine transplant model [9].

After extensive preliminary work, a system for the treatment of platelets was developed for use in human clinical trials. The system employed in clinical trials uses a platelet additive solution (Intersol—also known as PAS III) to dilute the platelet suspension to enhance pathogen inactivation. The platelets are treated and stored in a series of connected plastic containers developed by Baxter Healthcare Corporation (Round Lake, IL). Upon addition of S-59, the platelets are illuminated with 3 Joules/cm^2 of ultraviolet light for approximately 3 minutes with agitation. After illumination, the platelets are transferred to a final container which has a compound adsorption disc or CAD. This has previously been referred to as an S-59 reduction device or SRD. The purpose of the CAD is to reduce non-reacted S-59 and residual photo-product concentrations. The platelets are stored with the CAD for approximately 6 hours, then transferred to the final storage container. Upon transfer to the final storage container, the platelets are stored per current practice and may be used for transfusion.

The treatment system for plasma is essentially the same as that for platelets. Both platelets and plasma target 150 μM prior to illumination. The difference is that the plasma system uses a different final concentration of S-59. Thus, a blood bank would be able to prepare single unit pathogen-inactivated platelet and plasma components using the same UVA light device and similar disposable plastic containers. The length of the procedure is compatible with current preparation requirements of plasma and platelets.

After initial clinical studies in healthy subjects, it was necessary to obtain preliminary information on pathogen-inactivated platelets and plasma to determine their clinical efficacy. Additionally, the clinical trials to establish efficacy of pathogen-inactivated platelets and plasma have offered a renewed opportunity to rigorously examine the use of these components in medical practice. Quantitative data derived from prospective clinical trials is relatively rare in transfusion medicine as the introduction of blood components has been "grandfathered" into clinical practice and much of the use of blood component therapy is based on institutional practice with little evidence based data to support these practices [10,11].

Clinical trials of S-59 platelets

To assess the hemostasis efficacy of S-59 treated platelets, the first clinical trial in patients was conducted as a randomized, single blind crossover study where patients received either a sequence of S-59 treated platelets followed by Control platelets or Control platelets followed by S-59 platelets. Patients enrolled in the study were primarily bone marrow transplant patients who required support for their iatrogenic thrombocytopenia. The platelets were collected by apheresis. Hemostasis efficacy was evaluated by the use of the template bleeding time as well as clinical observation. That is, patients had a pre-transfusion bleeding time test and a post-transfusion bleeding time test at one and 24 hours after a study transfusion. Completion of the study required both an S-59 platelet transfusion and a control transfusion, each with its associated bleeding time observations. While the template bleeding time has been criticized for its lack of diagnostic specificity, it does provide an appropriate measure for a cohort of patients where hemostasis is the object of study. Secondary endpoints of the study included count increments and adverse events.

At study conclusion, the results demonstrated comparable shortening of the bleeding times. There was a slight difference in count increments that was not clinically significant. No adverse events were directly attributable to the S-59 platelets. Two larger studies in patients have been completed. They investigated the clinical efficacy of S-59 platelets. The first study (euroSPRITE), conducted in four European countries, examined the count increments as a primary endpoint using buffy coat-pooled platelets. The second study (SPRINT), conducted at 12 centers in the United States, has only recently been completed and the results are still being analyzed.

The euroSPRITE trial was initiated in 1998 and concluded in early 2000. One hundred and three patients were randomized and received either S-59 platelets (test) or platelets prepared in the standard manner (control). Patients received only study platelets for up to two cycles of support. Each cycle consisted of 56 days of transfusion support followed by 28 days of active surveillance. The primary endpoint of the trial was the platelet count increment one hour after transfusion with the analysis performed by longitudinal regression to account for the change in increments that have been reported in patients receiving platelets over several weeks. Secondary endpoints were such variables as the corrected count increment at one and 24 hours after transfusion and clinical measures of bleeding.

At the conclusion of the trial, there was no statistical difference in the one hour platelet increment between test and control cohorts. Similarly, there were no clinically significant differences between secondary endpoints such as interval between transfusion, refractoriness to platelet transfusion, adverse events and, significantly, RBC use. A second, larger multi-center trial (SPRINT) has recently been concluded (January 2001) in the United States. This trial enrolled over 600 patients, most of whom also were on oncological treatment regimens or were bone marrow transplant recipients. As with the European study, the trial was conducted in a double blind fashion; however, in contrast to the European study, approximately 50 pediatric patients were enrolled because the pre-clinical toxicology studies required for the admission of children into the study had been completed at the time of study initiation. While there were some design similarities with the euroSPRITE trial, this trial is distinguished by being the largest platelet trial to specifically examine the clinical efficacy of platelet transfusion. The primary endpoint of the study was a comparison of the proportion of study patients having grade 2 bleeding as defined by a World Health Organization bleeding scale. Grade 2 bleeding is primarily associated with chronic thrombocytopenia: prolonged oozing from cuts and mucocutaneous hemorrhage. This endpoint reflects the most statistically accessible concern in patients who require transfusion support with platelets. Secondary endpoints consisted of comparisons of the incidences of more serious bleeding (grades 3 and 4) as well as similar endpoints examined in the European study.

Patients in the SPRINT study were eligible to receive up to 28 days of study platelet support followed by a seven-day active surveillance period where they were examined for any adverse consequences of receiving study platelets. Following this, eligible patients could receive additional study platelet support in a second cycle (Figure 1).

Both the photochemical treated Test platelets and the standard Control platelets were prepared at the institutions participating in the trial. Other than the additional labor attendant to participating in the trial, there was little or no disruption in blood bank operations.

The trial enrolled 645 patients who received a transfusion from August 1999 through January 2001. Ninety-one patients received transfusion support beyond the 28 days by participating in Cycle 2. At the time of this conference (October,

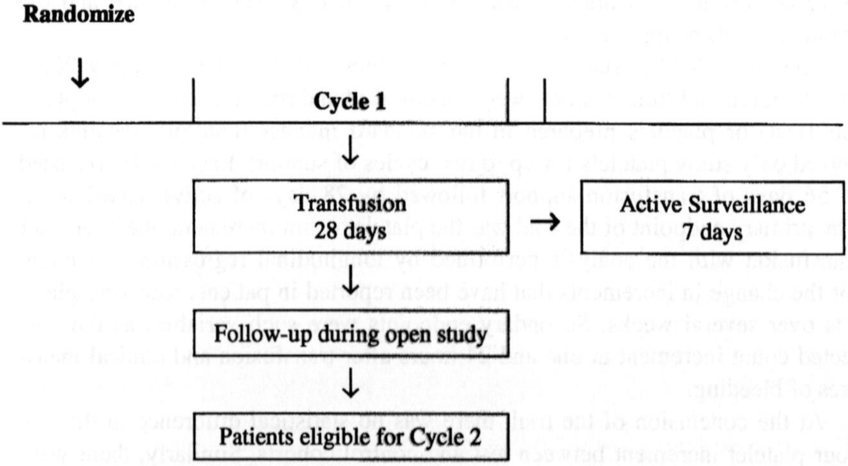

Figure 1. SPRINT study design mirrored clinical practice.

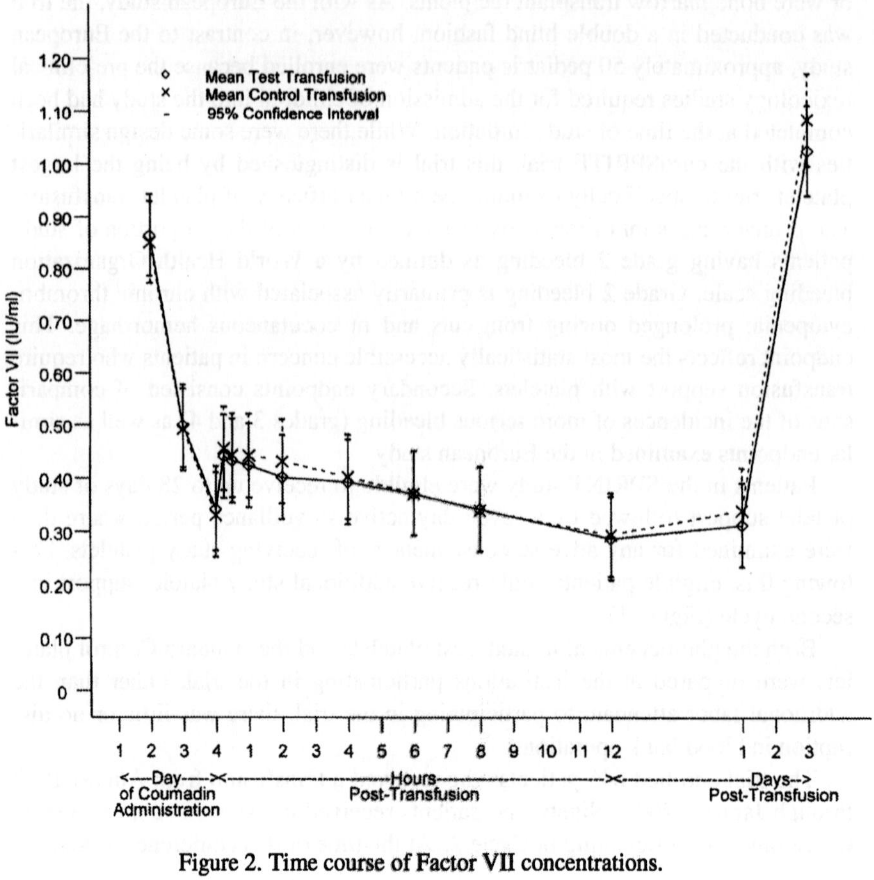

Figure 2. Time course of Factor VII concentrations.

2001), data from the trial are being reviewed, but sufficient data are available to demonstrate that there was no difference in the extent of grade 2 bleeding between the Test and Control groups of the trial. Final data are expected to be available later in 2001.

Studies of S-59 Plasma

There have been extensive clinical trials of S-59 plasma, running in parallel to the platelet studies described above. Of interest are a Phase 2 study, which is the first to have ever examined the pharmacokinetic properties of FFP, and a recently completed trial of 120 patients with acquired coagulopathy undergoing extensive surgical procedures such as liver transplantation. This latter trial is the largest prospective study conducted to examine the efficacy of plasma transfusions.

After an initial Phase 1 trial of S-59 FFP was completed in healthy subjects to establish preliminary tolerability, a second study was initiated to obtain detailed pharmacokinetic information inaccessible by in vitro studies. The Phase 2 study was conducted as a single blind, two period crossover study. Thirty subjects donated plasma over an average of six apheresis sessions. At each apheresis, plasma was prepared according to a standard procedure to serve as a control or to be treated with the S-59 pathogen inactivation process. Healthy subjects were then randomized to receive either a sequence of Test FFP followed by Control FFP or vice versa with a two-week minimum washout period between transfusions. For four days prior to each transfusion, subjects received 7.5 mg of Warfarin to iatrogenically lower their Factor VII levels. For the 24 hours following transfusion of the FFP, blood samples were taken for Factor VII measurements to determine the persistence and extent of Factor VII increments due to transfusion of study FFP. The crossover design of the study allowed for great statistical power to detect any differences in the pharmacokinetic variables of Factor VII in S-59 treated plasma compared to the Control plasma.

Twenty-seven subjects completed all apheresis sessions and transfusions. (Three subjects dropped out during or after the apheresis sessions without receiving a transfusion. This was due to inability in two subjects to tolerate apheresis and an unrelated adverse event in a third subject.) The time course of Factor VII concentrations from all 27 subjects are shown in Figure 2. As is apparent from the figure, there is essentially no difference in the results following S-59 FFP transfusion and standard (control) FFP transfusion. This is borne out by examination of the calculated pharmacokinetic variables for Factor VII in Test plasma and Control Plasma (Table 1). In addition to providing a detailed look at the properties of S-59 FFP, this study is significant for being the first rigorous evaluation of FFP transfusion of any kind.

Further extensive pharmacokinetic data on S-59 has been reported from an open label study of its use in the support of patients with rare congenital coagulation factor deficiencies [12]. Much like earlier studies reported on solvent detergent plasma [13], this trial was conducted as a single arm study where

Table 1. Calculated pharmacokinetic parameters of Factor VII (mean ± SD*)

Parameter	Test N=27	Control** N=27	p-value (Wilcoxon signed-rank test)
Half-life (hrs.)	3.3±2.8 median = 2.3	3.0±2.8 median = 19	.48
Clearance (mL/kg/hr)	39.0±57.1 median = 17.6	36.8±84.4 median = 16.4	.39
Recovery (% transfused)	43±17 median = 42	40±16 median = 43	.66
Volume of distribution (mL/kg)	142.9±73.8 median = 135.0	133.0±73.6 118.0	.65

* Standard deviation.

** Excluding three outliers, sequentially by Dixon's test (p<.005).

patients who required FFP for prophylaxis or treatment of bleeding received S-59 pathogen-inactivated FFP for up to a year. Other patients received an infusion of allogeneic plasma in a manner which allowed extensive pharmacokinetic measurement of their relevant missing factor in the transfused plasma. Eighteen patients with severe coagulation deficiencies of Factors I, II, V, VII, X, and XI were transfused as were members of a family with deficiencies of Protein C - the anticoagulation factor for which FFP transfusion may also be indicated.

Results from the study showed S-59 FFP provided hemostasis efficacy comparable to that shown in earlier transfusions the patients had received. Further, the adverse event profile of the S-59 FFP was similar to that seen for these patients prior to their enrollment in the study.

A larger clinical trial of S-59 FFP has recently (May, 2001) been completed. This prospective, two-arm, double blind study enrolled over 120 subjects who received either S-59 FFP (test) or standard FFP (control). After enrollment into the study, patients received only study FFP transfusions for seven days with an additional six-week follow up period to examine patients for long-term consequences of exposure to S-59 FFP. This trial was a study of safety as well as efficacy of S-59 FFP transfusion in patients undergoing invasive procedures such as liver transplantation. This was possible because the dose of FFP infused in this double blind trial was at the discretion of the treating physician. Some subjects have received over 70 units (approximately 17 liters) of S-59 FFP for the week they were on study. Approximately half of the patients received FFP in support of liver transplantation. As with the platelet trial, the data are currently being evaluated and are expected to be definitively reported in December 2001. However, analysis of the primary endpoint of the trial, a comparison of the ability of S-59 plasma to shorten the prothrombin time after transfusion with the ability of standard FFP showed no statistical difference. Data from this trial will be of general interest to the transfusion community because this is the first large prospective trial that has examined the use and efficacy of FFP in support of surgery.

A third trial of S-59 FFP is currently in progress. FFP is indicated for plasma exchange in support of patients with thrombotic thrombocytopenic purpura (TTP). In vitro studies have shown that S-59 FFP has no reduction in the von Willebrand Factor cleaving activity recently associated with TTP. As in a similar prospective, double blind trial conducted for solvent detergent plasma [13], this trial is one of the few prospective studies of the treatment of TTP. In other ways, this study has some important distinctions from the earlier solvent detergent plasma study and earlier studies of therapy for TTP. Specifically, the regimen of plasma exchange and concomitant medication is defined for both arms of the trial. Patients may receive either 40 or 60 mL/kg of plasma and a dose of 1 mg/kg of prednisone. The primary endpoint of the study is to compare the relapse rates (where relapse is defined as the return of thrombocytopenia or neurologic events) in those patients receiving S-59 FFP to the relapse rate of those receiving standard FFP in plasma exchange.

Trials of S-303-Treated RBCs

As mentioned earlier, development of a pathogen inactivation system for RBC concentrates has been more difficult because the viscosity and extremely high concentration of hemoglobin prevent the use of a light activated nucleic acid binding compound such as S-59.

As part of the expansion of Helinx™ technology, Baxter Healthcare and Cerus Corporation have also developed a non-light based approach to pathogen inactivation of RBC concentrates through the development and selection of a type of novel organic compound termed FRALE (Frangible Anchor Linker Effector). The selected FRALE, S-303, has a planar aromatic moiety which targets nucleic acids, and this moiety is, in turn, linked by an easily hydrolysable bond to a highly reactive alkylating moiety. Upon exposure to neutral pH conditions at room temperature, the S-303 either reacts with nucleic acids and prevents replication and transcription, or the linking bond hydrolyzes and the S-303 principally decomposes to an non-reactive negatively charged compound termed S-300 and a separate amino acid-like derivative. As in the S-59 photochemical process, a compound adsorption device is employed to reduce any remaining byproducts of the reaction, including S-300.

Extensive pre-clinical experiments have shown that the S-303 process is capable of inactivating high titers of both bacteria and viruses. Data have also been presented which show that leukocytes are inactivated by the treatment. In vitro properties of RBCs treated with the S-303 process demonstrate little or no difference in RBC hemolysis, potassium loss, morphology, and ATP concentrations as well as other RBC parameters of interest. Of equal importance, no changes were noted in RBC antigen typing. This significant issue was investigated further in the Phase 1B human study described below.

RBC preparation methods have historically been evaluated by a standardized procedure for determining recovery 24 hours after infusion into healthy subjects. Three trials have been completed in healthy human subjects to evaluate the recovery of autologous S-303 RBCs. The first two trials (Phase 1A and Phase 1B) did not incorporate the CAD as it was under development. The third trial, a

Table 2. Recoveries for each cohort

Study phase	Type RBCs	Number studied	% Recovery (± SD)
1A	Test (S-303 RBCs) single exposure	21	78.7±5.7
	Control	21	83.9±6.0
1B	Test (S-303 RBCs) These subjects had 4 total exposures	12	84.4±6.4
	Test (S-303 RBCs) These subjects had 5 total exposures	16	79.2±6.6

randomized crossover study, incorporated the CAD and the other components envisioned as part of the final treatment set. This trial examined the safety and tolerability of full unit S-303 autologous infusions as well as recovery 24 hours after infusion and RBC lifespan by continuing to follow the radiolabeled RBCs for 5 weeks after infusion.

The first trial, Phase 1A, was a single blind, two arm study in which 42 healthy subjects donated a unit of RBCs which was then treated with the S-303 process (Test) or was untreated (Sham Control). Sham treated RBCs were subjected to the same process parameters as Test RBCs, but without S-303 or Glutathione (GSH) addition, as Test RBCs. After thirty-five days of storage at 4°C, an aliquot of the RBCs was radiolabeled with 51-Cr according to established procedures [14]. The aliquot of radiolabeled cells was injected and samples were taken from the subject over the following 24 hours to determine recovery. Twenty-one subjects were in each arm of the study, and the results showed comparable recoveries (78.7% recovery for Test and 83.9% recovery for the Control). Significantly, both recoveries were above the 75% recovery expected for efficacious RBC preparations [15].

A particular concern of any RBC pathogen inactivation process is whether such treatment would alter the immunological profile of treated RBCs. While many patients receive RBCs over a short period of time for trauma, a substantial fraction of patients receive RBCs for periods of months to years. Creation of a "neoantigen" that could result in a hemolytic immune response after multiple infusions of pathogen inactivated RBCs would make any such system useless.

To investigate this possibility, a second recovery study (Phase 1B) was carried out using some of the same subjects who participated in the first recovery study. The Phase 1B trial was designed to evaluate whether multiple infusions of autologous S-303 treated RBCs resulted in an immune response to any hypothetical "neoantigens." The study was conducted as a single arm, open label study. Twenty-eight of the original 42 subjects participated in this second study. All subjects donated a full unit of RBCs which was then treated with the S-303 process (without the CAD). Then, at day 7, 14, 21, and 35 after donation, all subjects received a 10-30 mL aliquot of autologous S-303 RBCs. At day 35, the aliquot was again labeled with 51-Cr to determine recovery at 24 hours. In addition, before each infusion, a cross-match was done to detect any antibodies to the S-303 RBCs that might be circulating in the subject's serum. The results are shown in Table 2.

To fully appreciate the data, it is important to recognize at the conclusion of the Phase 1B trial that there were two cohorts of subjects: Sham/S-303 and Test S-303/S-303. One cohort received the Sham Control S-303 in the first trial and S-303/S-303 RBCs in the second. A second cohort received S-303 RBCs in the first trial, and S-303 RBCs in the second trial. The interval between trials was approximately 5 months, so the S-303/S-303 cohort had exposure to a total of five autologous S-303 RBC cell infusions over half a year.

Table 2 demonstrates that the recoveries for each cohort were consistent over time. There was no difference between the average recovery for subjects who received S-303 RBCs in the second study and their average recovery in the first study (control/S-303 cohort). These data suggest that there is no alteration in the immunological appearance of S-303-treated RBCs and that there is minimal or no effect of S-303 treatment on RBC recovery 24 hours after transfusion.

As mentioned previously, both of these studies were performed where the S-303 treatment process did not incorporate the compound adsorption disc (CAD). Further, in these studies, subjects received only a small aliquot of S-303-treated RBCs. To investigate the effect of the CAD on RBC circulation and to obtain tolerability and safety data, a third Phase 1 trial, (Phase 1C) was carried out. This trial was recently completed, and only preliminary data are available.

The Phase 1C trial consisted of two parts. Part A was a randomized, two period crossover study in which subjects received an aliquot of 51-Cr labeled S-303 RBCs (where the treatment employed the CAD incubation step) and RBCs prepared and stored in Adsol™ preservation solution (AS-1 RBCs) as the Control. Thus, in contrast to the two earlier studies, the Test RBCs represent the expected final configuration of the pathogen inactivation process and the Control cells represent current standard practice of RBC preparation. Furthermore, RBC life span (survival) was measured in addition to recovery 24 hours after transfusion. Life span measurements are not typically performed for RBC preparation methods, and there is less consensus on how best to measure life span [16].

The second part of the Phase 1C study, Part B, was conducted as a open label safety and tolerability study where 11 subjects received a full unit (~250 to 300 mL) of autologous 35-day-old S-303 RBCs. A panel of clinical laboratory assays as well as a physical examination with vital signs were obtained before and after the transfusion. Initial results from the study suggest that the full unit infusions were generally well tolerated and that the recovery of the S-303 RBCs was above 75%. Initial comparisons of recovery and life span data show no meaningful differences [17]. Final results of this study should be available at the end of 2001.

Conclusion

Clinical trials of blood components treated with pathogen inactivation systems have progressed to the point where it seems clear these trials can be a complementary method to maintain and enhance the safety of the blood supply. Solvent Detergent-treated plasma has been in use for over a decade in Europe and has recently been introduced into the United States. This method, however, requires pooling of plasma before treatment. Nucleic acid targeted methods of pathogen inactivation exemplified by the Helinx™ technology approach do not require pooling and allow for inactivation of non-enveloped viruses as well as bacteria and leukocytes. Platelets and plasma treated with Helinx™ technology using S-59 have been investigated in prospective randomized clinical trials. The results of these trials indicate that the photochemically-treated platelets and plasma show similar clinical efficacy as standard, untreated components. There are very promising data on the recovery and life span of RBCs treated with pathogen inactivation systems. Since RBC physiology is extremely well characterized, it is likely these promising results will be confirmed in patient studies. These data suggest that pathogen inactivation technology can be employed to enhance transfusion safety.

References

1. Goodnough LT, Brecher ME, Kanter MH, AuBuchon JP, Transfusion Medicine: First of Two Parts; N Engl J Med 1999;340:438-47.
2. Ling AE, Robbins KE, Brown TM et al. Failure of routine HIV-1 tests in a case involving transmission with preseroconversion blood components during the infectious window period. JAMA 2000;284:238-40.
3. Schuttler GC, Caspari C, Jursch CA, Gerlich WH, Schafer S. Hepatitis C virus transmission by a blood donation negative in nucleic acid amplification tests for viral RNA. Lancet 2000;355:41-42.
4. McDonald CP, Hartley S, Orchard K, et al. Fatal Clostridium perfringens sepsis from a pooled platelet transfusion. Transfusion Med 1998;8:19-22.
5. Chiu EKW, Yuen KY, Lie AKW et al. A prospective study of symptomatic bacteremia following platelet transfusion and its management. Transfusion 1994;34:950-54.
6. AuBuchon JP, Birkmeyer JD, Busch M. Safety of the blood supply in the United States: opportunities and controversies. Ann Int Med 1997;127: 905-09.
7. Lin L, Cook DN, Wiesehahn GP, et al. Photochemical inactivation of viruses and bacteria in platelet concentrates by use of a novel psoralen and long-wavelength ultraviolet light. Transfusion 1997;37:423-35.
8. Corten L, Wiesehahn GP, Smyers JM et al. Photochemical inactivation of hepatitis B (HBV) and Hepatitis C (HCV) viruses in human plasma as assessed in a chimpanzee infectivity model. Blood 2000;96:Supplement 1.
9. Grass JA, Wafa T, Reames A, et al. Prevention of transfusion-associated graft-versus-host disease by photochemical treatment. Blood 1999;93:3140-47.

10. Gmur J, Burger J, Schanz U, Fehr, Schaffner A. Safety of a stringent prophylactic platelet transfusion policy for patients with acute leukemia. Lancet 1991;338:1223-26.
11. Weiskopf, R. Do we know when to transfuse red cells to treat acute anemia? Transfusion. 1998;38:517-21.
12. deAlarcon P, Benjamin R, Shopnick M et al. An open-label trial of Fresh Frozen Plasma (FFP) treated by the Helinx™ single-unit photochemical pathogen inactivation system in patients with congenital coagulation factor deficiencies. Blood 2000;96 supplement 1:254.
13. Inbal A, Epstein O, Blickstein D, Kornbrot N, Brenner B, Martinowitz U. Evaluation of solvent/detergent treated plasma in the management of patients with hereditary and acquired coagulation disorders. Blood Coag Fibrinolysis. 1993;4:599-604.
14. Moroff G, Sohmer PR, Button LN et al. Proposed standardization of methods for determining the 24-hour survival of stored red cells. Trans-fusion 1984;24:109-14.
15. Heaton, WAL. Evaluation of posttransfusion recovery and survival of transfused red cells. Transfusion Med Reviews 1992;6:153-69.
16. Lotter G, Rabe W, de Lange A, et al. Reference values for red cell survival times. J Nucl Med 1991;32:2245-48.
17. Rios J, Hambleton J, Viele M, et al. Helinx™ treated RBC transfusions are well tolerated and show comparable recovery and survival to control RBCs. Transfusion. 2001;41:supplement 38s.

GCBS, ICBS AND OTHER INITIATIVES – THE *PARS PRO TOTO* PHENOMENON; WILL THERE EVER BE A *TOTUM PRO PARTE*?

Cees Th. Smit Sibinga[1]

Introduction

Blood transfusion is one of the routes for transmission of disease. Prevention of such transmission depends primarily on structure and organisation of the blood supply from vein to vein, the human resources involved and their education and training as well as their authority, responsibility and accountability. Above all it depends on the implementation and functioning of a quality system and quality management. Key elements are leadership at any level in the organisation, human resources and quality awareness.

Since the United Nations in 1948 formally declared in writing the human rights [1] with health, education and shelter for all as the elementary factors, a number of initiatives has been developed such as the 1975 World Health Assembly (WHA) adopted global programme 'Health for all by the year 2000' [2] and the 1988 institution of the Global Blood Safety Initiative (GBSI) [3], a joint effort of the World Health Organisation (WHO), the International Red Cross (IRC), the International Society of Blood Transfusion (ISBT) and the World Federation of Hemophilia (WFH). The latter initiative specifically focused on the safety and sustainability of the blood supply on national level through a global approach, triggered by the devastating AIDS epidemic.

In 1994 a global summit on AIDS was organised in Paris, where it was accepted that blood safety should be given a much higher priority on the top list of initiatives and it was proposed to approach this initiative through global collaboration of the manifold of organisations, whether governmental or non-governmental – Global Collaboration for Blood Safety (GCBS) [4]. This uniting initiative was supported by the adopted resolution WHA 48.27 during the 48th WHA in 1995 [5]. However, it lasted until late 2000 before the first gathering of the parties involved took place in Geneva at the WHO Headquarters. In 1998 a group of leading scientists from the medical and health sciences field together with some prominent virologists and transfusion medicine specialists decided to create another initiative, the International Consortium on Blood Safety (ICBS) [6]. This initiative was created because of dismay with the barely existing safety and efficacy of the blood supply that exists in most restricted economy countries

1. Director WHO Collaborating Center for Blood Transfusion and Sanquin Consulting Services, Blood Bank Noord Nederland, Groningen, NL. Vice-president, AABB Consulting Services Division, Groningen, NL.

as opposed by the high level of safety and efficacy in the industrialised countries. In 1999 WHO initiated the prestigious global Quality Management Programme (QMP) [7].

All these initiatives have as a common denominator a focus on safety, efficacy, sustainability and rational use of the blood supply, whether local, national or international. Certainly much has been done and achieved over the last few decades of the 20th century. However, even more is still to be done to provide health, education and the creation of awareness, as well as the set up of structure and organisation in the blood supply.

A fact is that today there are astonishing differences in vein to vein quality, quantity and availability of the blood supply within the member states of the United Nations despite the declaration of human rights in 1948 and the launching of the global programme 'Health for all by the year 2000' in 1975.

Lessons learned

Despite all initiatives created, launched and adopted in various meeting and conference rooms around the world, lessons have been learned during these last few decades of the 20th century. All these promising and often marvellous initiatives, which involved dozens of experts and dedicated professionals from all over the world, however, turned out to be insufficiently effective and inefficient because of the old and experienced '*pars pro toto*' principle.

What lessons have been learned that could be used to come to more effective and efficient endeavours?

In the first place it became evident that success depends on people, not on paper - the creation of true awareness at all levels, commitment and involvement, the acceptance of obligation and responsibility and the development of real ownership;

Second, soloist endeavours whether institutional or individual are bound to fail – only Atlas was able to carry the world on his shoulders, but that has never ever been duplicated since then;

Third, based on the declaration of Human Rights health and therefore health care has become a national affair, political awareness and commitment are crucial.

As a number four lesson it became clear that money and materialistic support are indeed important, but not crucial to the development of safe and sustainable blood supply systems where additionally it became evident that systems of what ever nature only function when appropriately managed. Management is an intellectual process privileged to the human being, to what is in between the human ears.

Who are the major players in the field?

There are many organisations in the world that have developed initiatives and programmes focused on the prevention of spread of infectious diseases through blood transfusion. Among these are some major players:

World Health Organisation (WHO) - Following the outbreak of the AIDS epidemic, WHO launched the Global Programme on AIDS (GPA) [8] under the dynamic leadership of Dr. Jonathan Mann. Over the first few years it became evident that an important route for spread of the virus was through contaminated blood donated for transfusion.

Global Blood Safety Initiative (GBSI) [3]

Although the spread through blood transfusion was only a 6 to 10% of the total spread, the outcome of a contaminated blood transfusion is almost invariably fatal. In 1988 it was therefor decided to create a separate initiative focused exclusively on the transfusion issue. This initiative was a first joint endeavour of 4 major organisations interested in a safe and sustainable blood supply – WHO, the then League of Red Cross and Red Crescent Societies (LRCRCS), the International Society of Blood Transfusion (ISBT) and the World Federation of Hemophilia. The core group of this Global Blood Safety Initiative (GBSI) was composed of expert representatives of each of these four organisations – Dr. W. Nigell Gibbs for the WHO Department of Laboratory Technology, Dr. Anthony H.F. Britten for the Blood Transfusion Department of the LRCRCS in Geneva, Dr. Bahman Habibi from Paris for the ISBT and Dr. Cees Th. Smit Sibinga from Groningen for the WFH. GBSI focused on assessing the current situation in the world, planning action and facilitating implementation of safe and sustainable blood supply systems all over the world. The outcomes of the various meetings and projects were a series of valuable recommendations and guidelines addressing the most urgent situations and needs in the world.

Blood Safety and Clinical Technology (BSCT)

Following a restructuring within WHO blood safety together with clinical technology issues became part of the Pharmaceuticals and Health Technology Cluster in 1998. Dr. Jean Emmanuel, former medical director of the Zimbabwe Red Cross Blood Transfusion Service in Harare, became director of the department and managed to create a competent staff in particular for the complex blood safety issues. Apart from the initiative to design specific distance learning materials for the various aspects in blood transfusion such as donor issues, testing and component production, an Aide Mémoire on Blood Safety [9] was put together covering four major principles: 1. National structuring and organisation of the blood supply; 2. voluntary and non-remunerated blood donation. 3. Testing of all collection, and 4. Appropriate clinical use of blood and blood components, that should serve as a simple guideline for the institution of safe, efficacious and sustainable blood supply. During a major consultation in Geneva of blood transfusion experts and directors of Collaborating Centers is was strongly advocated to add a fifth binding principle to the four elements of the Aide Mémoire – quality management. This was in 1999 the starting signal to the creation of a major and prestigious global project: Quality Management Programme (QMP) [10] to be implemented through structured and uniform Quality Management Training courses to be organised in each of the six WHO regions of the world.

A core group of expert advisors and consultants was formed to construct the programme and design the teaching and training curriculum and materials.

Because of the urgent need for action in Africa a first course was organised in Harare, Zimbabwe for a selected number of anglophone African countries in September 2000. In 2001 blood safety was accepted as the number seven top priority of WHO.

Global Collaboration on Blood Safety (GCBS) [4] - In 1994 the Global Blood Safety Initiative came to a formal end during the Paris AIDS summit, where blood transfusion safety was selected as a major priority. As a consequence the need for a more structured global collaboration to improve blood safety was discussed. Prime motives were the need to build on knowledge, utilising more efficiently existing experience, promoting dialogue and suggesting more realistic, effective and practical mechanisms to improve safety of the blood supply. The outcome was a proposal to create a Global Collaboration on Blood Safety (GCBS). In 1995, this proposal was brought to the notice of the 48th World Health Assembly, which after discussion adopted resolution WHA48.27 supporting the principles of a global collaboration on blood safety. Objective: to promote and strengthen international collaboration on safety of blood products and transfusion practices. Despite the urgent need for such international collaboration it lasted until late 2000 before a first constituting meeting of parties involved and interested was called to order by the then formed Department of Blood Safety and Clinical Technology (BSCT; Dr. Jean C. Emmanuel, director) of the WHO cluster on Pharmaceuticals and Health Technology (Dr. Suzuki, director). The mission of GCBS was formulates as follows: To improve collaboration among organisations and institutions involved in the area of transfusion safety, with a view to:

- encouraging and facilitating information exchange;
- promoting standards for GMP for blood related products for transfusion;
- fostering the establishment and implementation of co-operative partnerships to ensure donor and recipient safety in all countries.

Participants in this first constitutional meeting of GCBS were the American Association of Blood Banks (AABB), the European Plasma Fractionators Association (EPFA), the Féderation International des Organisations des Donneurs de Sang bénévole (FIODS), the International Federation of Red Cross and Red Crescent Societies (IFRCRCS), the International Pharmaceutical Plasma Industries Association (IPPIA), the World Federation of Hemophilia (WFH), WHO, representatives from developing countries, the health industry and prescribers.

There were also observers invited from the European Union (EU), the Council of Europe (CoE), the American Food and Drugs Administration (FDA) and National Institutes of Health (NIH), and the International Consortium on Blood Safety (ICBS). To elaborate a plan of action and address key issues three working groups were formed during the meeting:

- working group on quality assessment and assistance for development;
- working group on the policy process;
- working group on plasma issues.

International Consortium on Blood Safety (ICBS) - Because of dismay with the high level of blood safety and efficacy in industrialised countries that barely exists in most restricted economy countries Dr. Alfred Prince from New York Blood Center together with a group of leading blood bankers, virologists and public health experts in 1998 founded the International Consortium on Blood Safety (ICBS) [6]. The goals formulated are

- to identify, validate and make available high-quality affordable tests and test kits for HBV, HCV and HIV;
- to develop quality control and quality assurance programmes for laboratory testing;
- to co-ordinate technology transfer and to develop regional test kit manufacturers;
- to co-ordinate with other international organisations and professional societies providing educational support to improve donor selection and rational clinical use of blood;
- to foster collaboration with WHO and other relevant international organisations, professional and scientific societies.

Based on these goals specific objectives were formulated:

- to assess currently available TTI screening kits for costs, sensitivity and specificity;
- to obtain funding for targeted projects;
- to support national projects and do Demonstration Projects in developing countries to achieve universal blood safety by 2005;
- to maintain and strengthen liaison with WHO and other international organisation, professional and scientific societies;
- to sponsor regional workshops on quality assurance and Good Laboratory Practices and education in screening technology, donor management and rational clinical use of blood.

The Consortium has a limited number of full members and an important group of liaison members from most of the active national and international organisations, professional and scientific societies as well as patient organisations in the world involved and committed to blood safety (table 1). The group has formulated four major strategies to accomplish its goals:

- Support of National projects:
- assist in test evaluation and licensing by furnishing fully characterised test panels to national authorities;
- advice on efficient procurement mechanisms;
- play a role in training by offering 'train the trainer' workshops to assess performance of TTI screening in the field;
- assist in establishing national confirmatory laboratories.
- Assessment missions:
- assessment of current situation where countries express a need;
- report on these assessments with a Plan of Action;
- establish a Memorandum of Understanding with Health Authorities;
- co-ordinate project proposals and action/implementation;
- set indicators for monitoring and evaluation.

- Conduct Demonstration Projects:
- – identification and evaluation of high-quality affordable tests for HBV, HCV and HIV;
- – use selected reagents (kits) to assure all blood is tested in the project area;
- – include all BTSs, large and small;
- – assure quality of performance (consistency);
- – expand the programme over various regions and countries;
- – foster bulk purchase to assure continued affordability and availability;
- – foster improved criteria for donor selection and rational clinical use;
- Build network:
- – liaise with WHO and other relevant professional and scientific organisations and societies
- – participate in national and international projects;
- – create trust and confidence;
- – offer expertise and knowledge;
- – co-operate where possible and requested.

For the initial projects ICBS received funding from the Bill and Melinda Gates Foundation.

Who else are players in the field?

World Bank (WB) - has prioritised funding on a soft loan basis for national projects related to blood safety in restricted economy countries and actively seeks for expert advice and implementation of such projects

Council of Europe (CoE) and European Union (EU) – have developed programmes to foster and support projects for developing blood safety in restricted economy countries, both inside and outside Europe. The main emphasis of these programmes is on HIV and related TTI testing and on organisation and structuring of the blood supply. Projects are usually offered as a tender to consulting agencies for expertise and implementation.

Other players in the field – there are many interested parties such as

- patient organisations: e.g. World Federation of Hemophilia (WFH) , Thalassaemia International Federation (TIF)
- national professional organisations: the Netherlands SANQUIN Blood Supply Organisation and the American Association of Blood Banks (AABB) offering expertise and systems for implementation through expert consulting services focused on advice, teaching and training, technical support, reference functions, etc..
- Swiss Red Cross, offering financing of projects focused on organisation, structure of national blood supply systems, equipment and facilities.

The listing of players in the field is by far complete, as many other non-governmental organisations (NGOs) structured or just as it comes along with other projects and interests, exist.

Major questions to be answered

Over the past decades much attention has been given to the issue of blood safety, nationally and internationally. However, the national interest has been more concentrated in the industrialised world rather than in the restricted economy world where the problems related to unsafe blood are substantially bigger with a noticeable lack of awareness and commitment at virtually every level. Despite all the internationally developed initiatives only modest progress has been made due to the complexity of structuring and developing national health care systems in countries where education and economy suffer from poorly developed infrastructure of any kind. Despite all the major and other players in the field of blood safety, all the experts and consultants, major questions have to be answered to allow the designing of possible solutions to reduce further spread of infectious diseases through blood transfusion and develop truly effective preventive systems and management.

- How to create true and sustainable co-operation and collaboration on a global scale and level?
  This question certainly relates to the need to identify potential leadership and management, motivated and sufficiently experienced, committed, broad minded and with vision.
- How to effectively and professionally co-ordinate the many projects, requests and resources - both human and financial, to allow real action and completion of goals and missions to take place?
  This question relates to the need for a global database and clearinghouse as well as the need for clear selection criteria for an optimal and rational use of human and financial resources available.
- How to change the still ineffective *pars pro toto*, the attitude of various players in the field to claim the projects, support and resources as exclusive expert organisations into an effective *totum pro parte*, a true co-operation and collaboration in which each of the players complementary contributes to satisfactory and sustainable outcomes as expected, well monitored and evaluated?

These questions are to be answered in an open discussion between the players in the field before further actions, initiatives and projects are undertaken. Conference hall collaboration and co-operation become just facades when there is no structure of co-operation and collaboration, respected and visionary leadership and and a culture of mutual respect and confidence.

Possible solutions

What direction should we go to come to a baseline acceptable and affordable safety and efficacy of blood transfusion, irrespective of what hospital bed a patient is in?

Possible solutions or at least elements for a solution are in

- the organisation of an effective and up to date communication network;
- joint efforts: collaboration in stead of competition;

- mutual confidence, respect and co-operation as key elements of successful teamwork;
- respecting each others limitations, weaknesses and restrictions;
- respecting each others strengths, expertise, specific knowledge and experience;
- open exchange of experience.

There are more elements to think of such as wisdom, flexibility and sense of humour that could contribute.

Whatever direction the solution moves, the leading factor in the prevention of transmissible diseases through blood transfusion should be the common goal – a universal (global) safe, efficacious and sustainable blood supply available and affordable to each and every citizen in the world based on the WHO Aide Mémoire principles:

- National structures and organisation through political awareness and commitment;
- Reliable and repeat donor populations, established through appropriate public awareness, from low risk sections of the community, voluntary and non-remunerated;
- Reliable TTI testing of all donations for at least HBV, HCV, HIV and syphilis;
- Quality management through an optimal use of human and financial resources, creating professional awareness and ownership among all personnel.

However, the key factor is **leadership**.

References

1. United Nations Declaration of Human Rights, New York, NY, 1948.
2. WHO WHA30.43 1978: Declaration of Alma-Ata: Health for All by the Year 2000.
3. Report of the Global Blood Safety Initiative, WHO/GPA.DIR/88.9, Geneva 1988.
4. Report of the first meeting of the Global Collaboration for Blood Safety. WHO/BTS/01.1, Geneva 2001.
5. WHO WHA95 48.27 resolution, Geneva 1995.
6. International Consortium for Blood Safety. www.icbs-web.org.
7. WHO/BCT Quality Management Program, Geneva 2000.
8. WHO Global Program on AIDS, Geneva 1983.
9. WHO BTS Aide Mémoire on Blood Safety, Geneva 1999.

DISCUSSION

Moderators: R.Y. Dodd and H.J.C. de Wit

R.Y. Dodd (Rockville, MD, USA): Now we have some time for a broad discussion, focussing largely on the presentations that have been made this morning. Actually I like to lead it off by asking for a little debate between Dr Wages and Dr. Smit Sibinga on the potential role of pathogen inactivation as a means to solving some of the developing world's problems with transfusion transmissible infections. Dr. Wages, what do you think?

D.S. Wages (Concord, CA, USA): Thanks Dr. Dodd. I think your question is a good one. We often get asked about this. One question that I was asked in a meeting, I actually stumbled over, – was why doesn't one use a compound which works on red cells, also for platelets and plasma. The answer to that is that you can't get good pathogen inactivation to the high degree, that would be necessary for a truly efficacious method of pathogen inactivation using just one compound. I raise that because as Dr. Smit Sibinga mentioned, in many countries blood components are hard to get access to and just being able to obtain whole blood is an important issue. Right now the technology of pathogen inactivation has been engineered to address specific blood components. We do not as yet, have a system or a compound that can treat whole blood which can than be separated into a ten individual components. So, what the issue is, is that the current status of pathogen inactivation requires and presupposes the existence of a blood component preparation technology and infrastructure. Now, that can happen in various countries, but right now at least, for pathogen inactivation one has to have an infrastructure that is dedicated to preparing blood components before you can have effective pathogen inactivation.

C. Th. Smit Sibinga (Groningen, NL): Well, I am glad you mention that. Because, one has to build one's house starting with the foundation and not with the rooftop, let it be by starting with the decoration from the inside. What I re-iterate here again is the need for structure and organization. Building up an infrastructure, creating awareness, the first thing that leads to at least availability before one looks into the next issue which is the putting in place a sustainable and consistent program focussed on the blood safety. So, basic testing, starting with that. If you bring in the sophistication as we do have at this point in time you fail. We have had the presentation on the NAT. Such technology can not be implemented properly in a situation where even basic power supply, electricity is not guaranteed. So, develop step by step. However, the essential issue that relates to it is the difference between the 'haves' and the 'don't haves'. Between those who are still struggling for survival, not only per day but even per part of a day, and those that think of how could we further polish up and get all the exiting sophistication working. There are therefore huge discrepancies still to bridge. Make the gap closer therefore, before implementing these technologies. I have been approached earlier this meeting, would it not be appropriate to just skip the whole development in this large part of the world that struggles with the development and implement right away pathogen activation, so you don't need to bother about all the testing, all the validation etc., etc. I think it is not appropriate, but maybe you have a different view. I sense that you don't have that different a view, but you may have.

D.S. Wages: No, in fact I do have a different view. I think, – in fact, that to me the benefit of pathogen inactivation in any system like that for preparation of blood components is that it does allow greater flexibility in how you maintain safety of a blood supply. I think it is unrealistic, and I will speak only to the United States, because that's the country I am the most familiar with, at least initially for safety to be maintained by a pathogen inactivation. Once introduced it could theoretically lead to and completely replace and remove the other aspects of maintaining safety. I think one can see that as a possibility. What do I mean by that? Well, specifically, there are a number of tests used to maintain safety based on screening donors such as the syphilis test and ALT, that are done on all blood donors. The sensitivity and specificity of those tests is relatively limited in terms of enhancing blood safety. If you had a pathogen inactivation plus all the other screening mechanisms, those tests really are probably redundant. Eventually I think you'll see as pathogen inactivation systems become employed, tests like that starting to be removed from the procedures for enhancing safety. If that occurs in countries like the United States, it is common sense to me at least for people to try to figure out where the best cost effectiveness will be in countries that may have to be a little more selective in how they spend money on enhancing transfusion resources. Probably, one thing where you get the best cost effectiveness would just be the donor interview. You probably get the largest amount of added safety there, but in some societies or some countries where you have to be more selective with your money and also just the prevalence of infectious rates as HIV, you may want to immediately go to a pathogen inactivation system, provided that you have the infrastructure for component preparation. Perhaps, depending again on what the individual circumstances imply in some screening tests versus not others. I think trying to come up with the 'one solution fits all' is probably not going to work. So again, having an additional method for enhancing blood supply safety such as pathogen inactivation increases the options that would be available to people.

R.Y. Dodd: All right, thank you. Two views. Are there any questions from the audience?

S.L. Stramer (Gaithersburg, USA): Just to continue that discussion. In a country where you have to set up all aspects of testing, not only for the major viral infectious agents, but for parasites or bacteria as well, it seems logical that if there were a possibility at a low cost to implement an inactivating agent that did not have a residual risk, that was efficacious and didn't have any safety concerns, that would be a simple approach that would hit a wide spectrum of agents and produce a relatively way of achieving safe blood supply. If you have a six and a half log inactivation of most viral agents, elimination of bacteria, protozoa and proteinaceous agents, it just seems like a simple and rational way to approach a safer blood supply, although, maybe idealistic

C.Th. Smit Sibinga: I think all of us agree on the concept. The problem, however, is that the implementation of the concept requires real well-developed infrastructure and that should be supported through a national structure and commitment. It also should have the guarantee for sustainability and that is where the discrepancy is. We are all together in a bias where the principle is fantastic and has a great potential. We talked about it last year during the 25th jubilee symposium where Dr. Corash launched a number of these principles[1]. But the other side of the coin is that basic infrastructure that guarantees economy, awareness, etc. When you get to that you have to set a plan with milestones, with indicators, with the monitoring and evaluation step by step to be developed. There are situations in the world where there are much higher priorities to be set and looked into then bringing in our advanced technology. So, if we set it as an ultimately reachable goal somewhere from here to the horizon – but as you know, when you approach a horizon it also moves further away – you never reach it. However, we do have to set certain goals and priorities in countries where the first needs are basic. Go for the simple technology so that at least a basic safety could be implemented. From there work our way up to further development and implementation of technology and sophistication. Than maybe, at a certain point in time – thinking of the first couple of decades to come – you could just jump over a number of stages that we had to go through in the Western world to develop our technology. If you look at the material which Dr. Dodd showed at the very beginning you might realize the short time frame since the late seventies and 2000, and the huge amount of test developments that we have implemented and how rapidly that had an impact on the increase of the safety. But still we are not satisfied, we want to be below zero risk even.

J.H. Marcelis (Eindhoven, NL): Dr. Smit Sibinga, you showed us the magnificent information of future good health system by save blood production all over the world. What struck me most was the sentence you said: " A realistic view on blood safety". I think that holds too for the developed countries. I wonder, how is the impact of the World Health Organization on for instance European community legislation. Is it possible that World Health Organization can influence the legislation on for instance European countries to stop making new laws for

1. Corash LM. Inactivation of viruses, bacteria, protozoa and leukocytes in labile blood componentrs by using nucleic acid targeted methods. In: Smit Sibinga CTh, Cash JD eds. Transfusion Medicine: Quo Vadis. What has been achieved, what is to be expected. Kluwer Acad. Publ, Dordrecht/Boston/London 2001:113-23.

continuing testing. So, can they stress on stopping developed countries doing useless tests like NAT?

C. Th. Smit Sibinga: Legislation and regulation is in the first place a political mechanism to come to structures in countries, ultimately defined by politicians, by cabinets, by parliaments, by ministers. WHO is a non-political organization. WHO works through governments and could recommend but never set certain standards, rules or regulations. You will not find a specific requirement that each and every country has to follow other than the principles laid down in the Declaration of Human Rights in 1948. There are the various resolutions but it is up to the individual country wherever on the world to think whether they should implement or not. If they don't, WHO can not force them into that. It is a non-political organization, which only can recommend. That is one of the weaknesses which is very clearly recognized within WHO. A lot can be done, but you need the willingness, the awareness, specifically on a political level in each and every member state. So, WHO could beat the drum and try to convince by recommending that there is a limit and that certain parts of our wealth should be shared and made available. But it is up to individual countries to decide whether they should or not. That is the situation – not realistic, but idealistic.

H.J.C. de Wit (Amsterdam, NL): It might be the moment to say some words about the Council of Europe, because the Council of Europe also plays a role in blood, blood politics and blood safety. But now at least for the European situation, there is a European Union Directive in preparation. These roles might change. Perhaps you could commend on that?

C.Th. Smit Sibinga: C.Th. Smit Sibinga: The Council of Europe also has already for quite some time blood safety as one of the top priorities for one of the departments. The department of Social Health, Mrs Gabriela Dragoni spoke about that last year in Groningen.[1] Also the Council of Europe, which has no real political power, makes recommendations. The European Union has a governing body which is called the Council of the European Union. The European Union could set Directives which overrule national legislation of the member states in the European Union. However, the Council of Europe could only recommend to all its 44 member states. The Council of Europe took initiative, a couple of years ago, to produce a Guide with a number of recommendations on the collection, the processing, the quality control and the use of human blood in hospitals, which now in its seventh edition.[2] That is a fantastic Guide because it provides a framework to many a country to be adopted in their own standards. I know of countries – you would be surprised if I name you one which is far away here but regarded to be a very developed and industrialized country, that is Australia. They did not reinvent the wheel, but they took the Guide of the Council of

1. Battaini-Dragoni G. Forword. In: Smit Sibinga CTh, Cash JD eds. Transfusion Medicine: Quo Vadis. What has been achieved, what is to be expected. Kluwer Acad. Publ, Dordrecht/Boston/London 2001:XI-XIII.
2. Guide to the preparation, use and quality assurance of blood components. 6th ed.CoE Publ. Strasbourg Cedex 2000.

Europe as their golden standard. So, that has an impact therefore. But the Council of Europe cannot set rules that overrule national legislation, unfortunately.

J.P.H.B. Sybesma (Dordrecht, NL): Dr. Wages, when do you think there would be a possibility that you could skip all the tests, the ELISA tests, the NAT test, the bacterial test? I don't know whether there would ever be a possibility, but it might be. I am not aware of the costs of your procedure. Of course it is much easier, you don't need to do all other tests. But would it be much cheaper when you skip all the tests and just inactivate? Do you think there is a possibility in a decade time that we can do that?

D.S. Wages: Thanks for the question. I think the best way to address that question is, that right now the cost is still not determined. Both the manufacturer such as Baxter Cerus Corporation are still trying to figure out what's the amount of money that they would like to get for this and what the market could afford. I always address to the question of how much it's going to cost by saying it will probably be somewhat less than what Baxter and Cerus want and somewhat more than people would like to pay. I know I will be right. But the answer to the question is that in theory it is quite possible. You could take a unit, not test it at all for the presence of virus, either by nucleic acid amplification techniques or the presence of antibodies and just treat it. This is why I made a point of this – whether that is the best approach is going to be somewhat dependent on the tolerance of risk of wherever this is occurring. For certain countries, the infrastructure for producing blood components at all is not even present, while there are certainly risks of getting transfusion transmitted infections. Let's remember, if you are in an automobile accident and you are bleeding to death, you got more pressing concerns. So, that is why I think the pathogen inactivation allows flexibility. I personally think along the lines of your question that you could certainly dispense with a lot of screening this way. I think for countries where there is a developed legal system, such as the United States, it would probably not be realistic for people to dispense with both aspects of safety at once. Because, inevitably, any pathogen inactivation technique is going to have failures, probably due to operator error or maybe a particular batch of S59 or the disposable is not adequately made. That is inevitable and if you are a patient you would like to have some sort of procedure to handle that. So, I think for a country like the United States, eventually many screening tests will probably be eliminated, but not all of them. For other countries there may be a shift where they jump immediately to pathogen inactivation once they have the infrastructure for component preparation.

J.H.P.B. Sybesma: So when you do not want to skip everything? Probably you can skip the NAT test and just keep the ELISA, in that way?

D.S. Wages: I think it would depend on the country and the amount of resources they want to spend to address the problem. Let us just assume you had a certain amount of money and you had to chose between pathogen inactivation system that worked – and again, this presupposes that you have the infrastructure for development of blood components – and conventional testing. So, now your question is, I can make blood components and I can decide, do I want to do screening or do I want pathogen inactivation. For many countries it probably might make more sense to just do pathogen inactivation.

H.J.C. de Wit: Which means that you have made a choice in the principal discussion whether you should start with the best raw material or make your refining process optimal. That is the principal question. But perhaps there is also a very practical, technical question in this debate: Is for all the expected viruses in whole blood, in the raw material anywhere in the world the inactivation procedure adequate to really inactivate some window donations such as for hepatitis C or other?

D.S. Wages: A good question. Talking about a pathogen inactivation system presupposes one of the things that I mentioned as being part of an ideal system, mainly that you get broad and robust pathogen inactivation. Now, in reality, the world is not quite that simple. There are some viruses where the S59 treatment system for example for platelets and plasma is able to inactivate extremely high titers, such as HIV. There are others where there is inactivation, but it is on several orders magnitude lower such as hepatitis A or Parvo-virus. Viruses that are very small and have extremely tight capsids are less susceptible to nucleic acid targeted methods of pathogen inactivation than larger enveloped viruses for example. Does that mean that they can not be eliminated? No, but I should point out at least in those two examples there are not methods for addressing them in current existence any way. That is why I personally think that probably the interview of the donor – much like in medical practice – just talking to the donor and getting a medical history is the cheapest and the most fundamental way of getting to the nature of the medical problem or in this case maintaining the safety of the blood supply.

C. Th. Smit Sibinga: Dr. Cuypers, in the advances of the technology you discussed certainly one end of the stick of development in further improving NAT testing etc. You even came up with the concept of the small minipool. The other end of the stick of development is focussed on the countries I pointed to, and that is in more sensitive and reliable, robust rapid tests. Have you any idea about what is going on, on that end of the stick where modern technology – biotechnology, microbiology and molecular biology – could be implemented in a simple robust rapid test with much higher sensitivity.

H.T.M. Cuypers (Amsterdam, NL): They are on their way, but also for the Western market for simple testing at home and similar applications. But I am not aware of thinking about very simple systems which are very cheap which then can be developed for the developing countries. Probably, of course there is not a commercial market for it, and most of the R & D work is done based on the market and not on the prospective of having better sales.

C.Th. Smit Sibinga: One should realise that if eighty percent of the world has no access -t that is a tremendous potential market.

H.T.M. Cuypers: Yes, but not a financial market.

H.J.C. de Wit: Could it be a solution to work in the more political world including WHO to a system where – when we realize that new systems due to patented systems are always very expensive – we come to a price policy such as has been introduced for anti-HIV drugs, which means that the Western world pays other prices than the developing world?

C.Th. Smit Sibinga: Certainly, that could be a mechanism.

H.T.M. Cuypers: What we saw from the press releases is that they are focussing on such a system that what we have to pay now in the West is not applicable to the developing countries including South-East Asia. But what the real financial benefits of are – you still have to pay for instance for an ELISA the price. Even we are paying very high prices already for ELISA for HIV, because they are ten times as expensive for HBV and HCV. Also in that type of test there is a lot of money for the intellectual property.

S.L. Stramer: Not to challenge the goals of ICBS, but hypothetically, in the evaluation of developing country tests, which are most likely simple, rapid tests, assuming a country fails the 200 member panel, then the country is left with nothing. Is part of ICBS policy to work with major world wide manufacturers of tests? Abbott and other companies are working with delivery systems to provide to the developing world dipstick methods that do not require water, that do not require electricity, that have limited amount of disposables. Will ICBS work with a test that could be developed for many countries rather than having thousands of independently developed tests that maybe substandard?

C.Th. Smit Sibinga: It is certainly one of the elements in the policy and therefore in the strategy of the ICBS, where one on the other side needs to be careful with also the ethical issues related to that. A lot of the development of the panel at the moment at CDC is done through collected and shipped voluntary donated plasma. So, there is the question of the ownership – will someone else go to the market to make money out of it where it was developed through the funding of the Bill & Melinda Gates Foundation for more idealistic purposes. How do you handle that? That is a matter which is currently being looked into through specific lawyers that know about these issues, to not really sell your soul to the devil. On top there is a dipstick that eventually still has a price that is not available.

R.Y. Dodd: Mr Adriani, yesterday we heard that screening for bacterial contamination is probably cost-effective on the broad health level. Could you tell me something very interesting about the cost-effectiveness of the process in your own center. I think it would be useful if you could answer the question. To what extent is this a value in your own practice?

W.P.A. van der Tuuk Adriani (Groniongen, NL): It is indeed a very interesting question. Many years ago the shelf life of platelets was seven days and it was reduced to five days due to a bacterial problem that was discovered at that time. Now, we have resolved this bacterial problem and we can extend the shelf life again to seven days. That means for at least our institute that the outdated product that we had to discard was decreased by ten percent at least. Before we extended our shelf life to seven days it was about twenty-five percent. Now it is ten to fifteen percent. So, those ten percent I can sell to the hospitals, it results in a saving as big as three hundred and fifty thousand guilders per year. When we subtract the cost of all the bacterial tests, which is about one hundred and fifty thousand guilders, we have a positive result of two hundred thousand guilders per year, which is a substantial amount of money.

R.Y. Dodd: Congratulations

J.H. Marcelis: I just want to add that it is not only money which you save, it is also all the fuss you have in the week-ends to have your platelets on emergency situations. If you add that to the costs you make, it is even better.

R.Y. Dodd: Dear friends, ladies and gentlemen, my task now is to close this symposium. In doing so, first I have to thank all of our speakers and moderators and our audience for their excellent work and very lively participation. Next, of course, we must thank Mr. Jansen van Galen for his hosting of this 26th Sanquin International Symposium, Mr. de Wit for his enthusiastic and continuing support of the process and all of the staff of the Blood Bank Noord Nederland who have done so much wonderful work, both behind the scenes and right here in front of us. Thank you so much.

But of course our greatest admiration and thanks go to Dr. Cees Smit Sibinga for his leadership and his own hard work in this 26th Symposium. During the meeting the concept of a diamond has come up from time to time and I think that this is one of the finest products of this wonderful country, the finished diamond. The diamond is really nothing until it is being turned into a jewel as result of the skill and indeed the courage of the cutter and polisher of the diamond. And it is in this role that I see Cees Smit Sibinga, lovingly polishing the rough symposium until the facets shine and cast light into a milliard of unexpected places. Over the past few days, this is precisely what has happened in this meeting. At first sight perhaps we were going to have in the rough what appeared to be a simple meeting on the status of infectious disease and transfusion. But, we have indeed heard the state of the art in this field and we have been reminded of risks to come, parasites and prions for example. But more importantly I believe, we have come to realize that this asymptotic search for zero risk comes at a disproportionate cost to the healthcare system (with the possible exception of bacterial screening). We must ponder the reasons for this strange truth that we are willing to put so many resources into so little gain. I think perhaps that Prof. Douglas Starr would have helped us here and I am confident that he will do so at some future symposium, here in Groningen. But I think too, we have been warned about what might be some unreal expectations that we have generated for ourselves as we think about what is to come. Pathogen inactivation as you have heard is just around the corner. Yet we learned at the same time in this symposium about the extraordinary fragility of the early embryo – indeed, before we even know there is an embryo there. Leading us, I think, to feel concern about the possible impacts of additives that will be necessary in order to inactivate blood products. Dr Wages himself commented that perhaps the promise of the next infectious agent to be inactivated is not quite as full as we hope it is. So, I get a little concerned when I hear an un-critical acceptance of these kinds of measures, particularly when undertaken by politicians. We also confidently and hopefully anticipate test for the pathologic form of the prion. Yet again, we heard that this might not be quite as easy as we had supposed. We really may not know what this test will mean and we may not know what the response of people will be to having to undertake this test to give blood. Remember that the risk factors for acquisition of a prion disease differ quite significantly from those from most of the other infections we have had to deal with. Certainly we started questioning donors and testing donors for HIV. But I think the significance of a positive test and the significance back to the donor's behavior were very much clearer in that circumstance.

Other new technologies may have a huge impact on patients' survival. We heard about xeno-transplantation, but we were cautioned about endogenous retroviruses which will be passengers in xeno transplants. What will their impact be? We really do not know it at this stage. Conversely, we were largely reassure that the genetic background of cord blood stem cell donors may not be as much of a concern as we had thought. But equally, the efficacy of this particular process may be limited, at least when used to treat inheritable metabolic diseases.

We have been reminded that the concept, the overriding concept of quality has been enthusiastically presented as a key to continued success. It is time to stop thinking that quality is something we have to endure in order to satisfy the regulators, but rather that we see it as a process to move us ahead in all of our endeavors wherever we are in the world.

I draw from this symposium three personal messages.

First, although it is very difficult to stare into the crystal ball in this arena, I think that today's problems in microbial safety have been solved in large part. At least in the Western world.

Second, now it is time perhaps to step back, review, re-simplify and rebuild. Remember the 650 year old lesson of William of Occam: 'Don't do with much, what can be done with little.' By contrast, and it is a strong contrast, I think that this reveals that we have been somewhat blind to the non-infectious hazards of transfusion. These issues have been raised and discussed but not in-depth at this meeting and I would like to think that one of your future meetings will focus on this area where the risks are greater than those that we now perhaps have come to grips with.

Finally, and I realize that my message is not entirely up beat, the contrast of what we do here in the developed world, with the situation in the developing world is staggering. How can we have been so selfish about our own safety and so totally ignore the rest of the world in our own professional specialty?

Thank you Dr. Cees Smit Sibinga, for setting up this chance for all of us to get together and allowing me to remind us that some of the shafts of light cast by the diamond are not always flattering and may indeed be painful. I would like again to thank everybody and to give Dr. Cees Smit Sibinga in particular my very best wishes for the next 24 symposia. A renewed thanks and goodbye to all.

INDEX

DEVELOPMENTS IN HEMATOLOGY AND IMMUNOLOGY

1. H.R. Lijnen, D. Collen and M. Verstraete (eds.): *Synthetic Substrates in Clinical Blood Coagulation Assays.* 1980 ISBN 90-247-2409-0
2. C.Th. Smit Sibinga, P.C. Das and J.O. Forfar (eds.): *Paediatrics and Blood Transfusion.* Proceedings of the 5th Annual Symposium on Blood Transfusion, organized by the Red Cross Blood Bank Groningen-Drenthe, The Netherlands (1980). 1982 ISBN 90-247-2619-0
3. N. Fabris (ed.): *Immunology and Ageing.* 1982 ISBN 90-247-2640-9
4. G. Hornstra: *Dietary Fats, Prostanoids and Arterial Thrombosis.* With an Introductory Chapter by A. Bleakley Chandler. 1982 ISBN 90-247-2667-0
5. C.Th. Smit Sibinga, P.C. Das and J.J. van Loghem (eds.): *Blood Transfusion and Problems of Bleeding.* Proceedings of the 6th Annual Symposium on Blood Transfusion, organized by the Red Cross Blood Bank Groningen-Drenthe (1981). 1982 ISBN 90-247-3058-9
6. J. Dormandy (ed.): *Red Cell Deformability and Filterability.* 1983 ISBN 0-89838-578-4
7. C.Th. Smit Sibinga, P.C. Das and H.F. Taswell (eds.): *Quality Assurance in Blood Banking and Its Clinical Impact.* Proceedings of the 7th Annual Symposium on Blood Transfusion, organized by the Red Cross Blood Bank Groningen-Drenthe (1982). 1984 ISBN 0-89838-618-7
8. A.M.H.P. van den Besselaar, H.R. Gralnick and S.M. Lewis (eds.): *Thromboplastin Calibration and Oral Anticoagulant Control.* 1984 ISBN 0-89838-637-3
9. P. Fondu and O. Thijs (eds.): *Haemostatic Failure in Liver Disease.* 1984 ISBN 0-89838-640-3
10. C.Th. Smit Sibinga, P.C. Das and G. Opelz (eds.): *Transplantation and Blood Transfusion.* Proceedings of the 8th Annual Symposium on Blood Transfusion, organized by the Red Cross Blood Bank Groningen-Drenthe (1983). 1984 ISBN 0-89838-686-1
11. H. Schmid-Schönbein, L.J. Wurzinger and R.E. Zimmerman (eds.): *Enzyme Activation in Blood-perfused Artificial Organs.* 1985 ISBN 0-89838-704-3
12. J. Dormandy (ed.): *Blood Filtration and Blood Cell Deformability.* 1985 ISBN 0-89838-714-0
13. C.Th. Smit Sibinga, P.C. Das and E. Seidl (eds.): *Plasma Fractionation and Blood Transfusion.* Proceedings of the 9th Annual Symposium on Blood Transfusion, organized by the Red Cross Blood Bank Groningen-Drenthe (1984). 1985 ISBN 0-89838-761-2
14. S. Dawids and A. Bantjes (eds.): *Blood Compatible Materials and their Testing.* 1986 ISBN 0-89838-813-9
15. C.Th. Smit Sibinga, P.C. Das and T.J. Greenwalt (eds.): *Future Developments in Blood Banking.* Proceedings of the 10th Annual Symposium on Blood Transfusion, organized by the Red Cross Blood Bank Groningen-Drenthe (1985). 1986 ISBN 0-89838-824-4
16. A. Berlin, J. Dean, M.H. Draper, E.M.B. Smith and F. Spreafico (eds.): *Immunotoxicology.* Proceedings of the International Seminar on the Immunological System as a Target for Toxic Damage – Present Status, Open Problems and Future Perspectives, in collaboration with the UNEP-ILO-WHO IPCS and the Commission of the European Communities. 1987 ISBN 0-89838-843-0
17. T. Ottenhoff and R. de Vries: *Recognition of M. leprae Antigens.* 1987 ISBN 0-89838-887-2
18. J.-L. Touraine, R.P. Gale and V. Kochupillai (eds.): *Fetal Liver Transplantation.* 1987 ISBN 0-89838-975-5
19. C.Th. Smit Sibinga P.C. Das and C.P. Engelfriet (eds.): *White Cells and Platelets in Blood Transfusion.* Proceedings of the 11th Annual Symposium on Blood Transfusion, organized by the Red Cross Blood Bank Groningen-Drenthe (1986). 1987 ISBN 0-89838-976-3
20. C.F.M. Hendriksen: *Laboratory Animals in Vaccine Production and Control.* 1988 ISBN 0-89838-398-6

DEVELOPMENTS IN HEMATOLOGY AND IMMUNOLOGY

21. C.Th. Smit Sibinga, P.C. Das and L.R. Overby (eds.): *Biotechnology in Blood Transfusion.* Proceedings of the 12th Annual Symposium on Blood Transfusion, organized by the Red Cross Blood Bank Groningen-Drenthe (1987). 1988 ISBN 0-89838-404-4
22. C.Th. Smit Sibinga, P.C. Das and C.F. Högman (eds.): *Automation in Blood Transfusion.* Proceedings of the 13th Annual Symposium on Blood Transfusion, organized by the Red Cross Blood Bank Groningen-Drenthe (1988). 1989 ISBN 0-7923-0488-8
23. S. Dawids (ed.): *Polymers: Their Properties and Blood Compatibility.* 1989 ISBN 0-7923-0491-8
24. C.Th. Smit Sibinga, P.C. Das and H.T. Meryman (eds.): *Cryopreservation and Low Temperature Biology in Blood Transfusion.* Proceedings of the 14th Annual Symposium on Blood Transfusion, organized by the Red Cross Blood Bank Groningen-Drenthe (1989). 1990 ISBN 0-7923-0908-1
25. C.Th. Smit Sibinga and L. Kater (eds.): *Advances in Haemapheresis.* Proceedings of the 3rd International Congress of the World Apheresis Association (Amsterdam, The Netherlands, 1990). 1991 ISBN 0-7923-1312-7
26. C.Th. Smit Sibinga, P.C. Das and P.M. Mannucci (eds.): *Coagulation and Blood Transfusion.* Proceedings of the 15th Annual Symposium on Blood Transfusion, organized by the Red Cross Blood Bank Groningen-Drenthe (1990). 1991 ISBN 0-7923-1331-3
27. C.Th. Smit Sibinga, P.C. Das and J.D. Cash (eds.): *Transfusion Medicine: Fact and Fiction.* Proceedings of the 16th International Symposium on Blood Transfusion, organized by the Red Cross Blood Bank Groningen-Drenthe (1991). 1992 ISBN 0-7923-1732-7
28. C.Th. Smit Sibinga, P.C. Das and T.H. The (eds.): *Immunology and Blood Transfusion.* Proceedings of the 17th International Symposium on Blood Transfusion, organized by the Red Cross Blood Bank Groningen-Drenthe (1992). 1993 ISBN 0-7923-2380-7
29. C.Th. Smit Sibinga, P.C. Das and H.J. Heiniger (eds.): *Good Manufacturing Practice in Transfusion Medicine.* Proceedings of the 18th International Symposium on Blood Transfusion, organized by the Red Cross Blood Bank Groningen-Drenthe (1993). 1994 ISBN 0-7923-3009-9
30. C.Th. Smit Sibinga, P.C. Das and E. Briët (eds.): *Hereditary Diseases and Blood Transfusion.* Proceedings of the 19th International Symposium on Blood Transfusion, organized by the Red Cross Blood Bank Groningen-Drenthe (1994). 1995 ISBN 0-7923-3694-1
31. C.Th. Smit Sibinga, P.C. Das and E.L. Snyder (eds.): *Trigger Factors in Transfusion Medicine.* Proceedings of the 20th International Symposium on Blood Transfusion, organized by the Red Cross Blood Bank Noord-Nederland (1995). 1996 ISBN 0-7923-4225-0
32. C.Th. Smit Sibinga, P.C. Das and B. Löwenberg (eds.): *Cytokines and Growth Factors in Blood Transfusion.* Proceedings of the 21th International Symposium on Blood Transfusion, organized by the Red Cross Blood Bank Noord-Nederland (1996). 1997 ISBN 0-7923-4787-0
33. C.Th. Smit Sibinga, P.C. Das and J.C. Fratantoni (eds.): *Alternative Approaches to Human Blood Resources in Clinical Practice.* Proceedings of the 22nd International Symposium on Blood Transfusion, organized by the Red Cross Blood Bank Noord Nederland (1997). 1998 ISBN 0-7923-8305-2
34. C.Th. Smit Sibinga and H.J. Alter (eds.): *Risk Management in Blood Transfusion: The Virtue of Reality.* Proceedings of the 23rd International Symposium on Blood Transfusion, organized by the Blood Bank Noord Nederland (1998).1999 ISBN 0-7923-6054-0
35. C.Th. Smit Sibinga and H.G. Klein (eds.): *Molecular Biology in Blood Transfusion.* Proceedings of the 24th International Symposium on Blood Transfusion, organized by the Blood Bank Noord Nederland (1999). 2000 ISBN 0-7923-6534-8
36. C.Th. Smit Sibinga and J.D. Cash (eds.): *Transfusion Medicine: Quo Vadis? What Has Been Achieved, What Is to Be Expected.* 2001 ISBN 1-4020-0079-0

MIX
Papier aus verantwortungsvollen Quellen
Paper from responsible sources
FSC® C105338

If you have any concerns about our products,
you can contact us on
ProductSafety@springernature.com

In case Publisher is established outside the EU,
the EU authorized representative is:
Springer Nature Customer Service Center GmbH
Europaplatz 3, 69115 Heidelberg, Germany

Printed by Libri Plureos GmbH
in Hamburg, Germany